HOUSE OFFICER
SERIES

Weiner & Levitt's

Pediatric Neurology

FOURTH EDITION

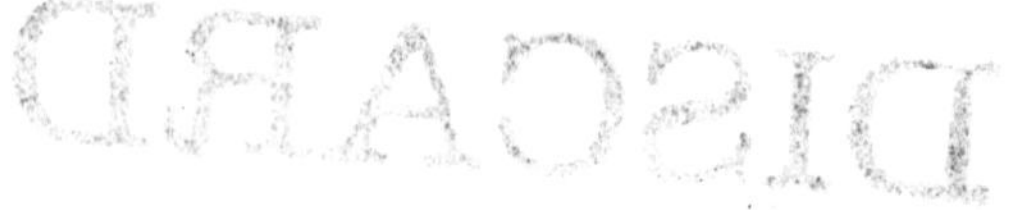

The House Officer Series is based on Weiner and Levitt's *Neurology for the House Officer*, first published in 1973.

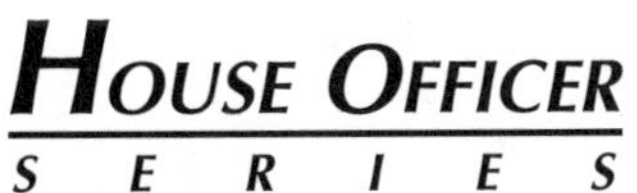

Weiner & Levitt's Pediatric Neurology

FOURTH EDITION

Michael E. Cohen, M.D.

Professor of Neurology and Pediatrics
The Children's Hospital of Buffalo
State University of New York at Buffalo
Buffalo, New York

Patricia K. Duffner, M.D.

Professor of Neurology and Pediatrics
The Children's Hospital of Buffalo
State University of New York at Buffalo
Buffalo, New York

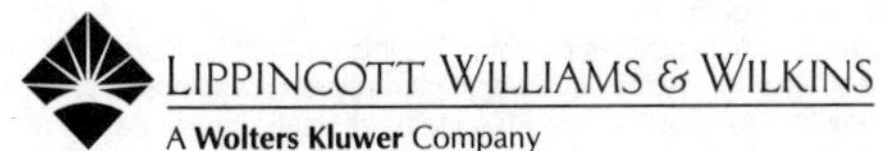

Philadelphia • Baltimore • New York • London
Buenos Aires • Hong Kong • Sydney • Tokyo

Acquisitions Editor: Charles W. Mitchell
Developmental Editor: Stacey L. Baze
Production Editor: Christiana Sahl
Manufacturing Manager: Benjamin Rivera
Cover Designer: Jeane Norton
Compositor: Circle Graphics
Printer: RR Donnelley/Crawfordsville

530 Walnut Street
Philadelphia, PA 19106 USA
LWW.com

Printed in the USA

Library of Congress Cataloging-in-Publication Data

Weiner & Levitt's pediatric neurology / Michael E. Cohen . . . [et al.].—4th ed.
p. cm. — (House officer series)
Includes bibliographical references and index.
ISBN 0-7817-2931-9
1. Pediatric neurology. I. Cohen, Michael E., 1937- II. Series.

RJ486.W35 2003
618.92'8—dc21

2002043458

Care has been taken to confirm the accuracy of the information presented and to describe generally accepted practices. However, the authors and publisher are not responsible for errors or omissions or for any consequences from application of the information in this book and make no warranty, expressed or implied, with respect to the currency, completeness, or accuracy of the contents of the publication. Application of this information in a particular situation remains the professional responsibility of the practitioner.

The authors and publisher have exerted every effort to ensure that drug selection and dosage set forth in this text are in accordance with current recommendations and practice at the time of publication. However, in view of ongoing research, changes in government regulations, and the constant flow of information relating to drug therapy and drug reactions, the reader is urged to check the package insert for each drug for any change in indications and dosage and for added warnings and precautions. This is particularly important when the recommended agent is a new or infrequently employed drug.

Some drugs and medical devices presented in this publication have Food and Drug Administration (FDA) clearance for limited use in restricted research settings. It is the responsibility of the health care provider to ascertain the FDA status of each drug or device planned for use in their clinical practice.

10 9 8 7 6 5 4 3 2 1

Dedication

To our spouses and all the students and residents
we have been privileged to train and to interact with over the years

Foreword

Pediatric Neurology was an outgrowth of the companion adult manual *Neurology*. The latter, first published in 1973, has gone through six editions and has been translated into eight foreign languages. Its "child," the pediatric manual, was inspired by the late Randolph K. Byers, a giant in the field of pediatric neurology in his generation. The pediatric manual was first published in 1977 with the invaluable assistance of Michael J. Bresnan, who likewise was key in the second edition. Michael Bresnan was a superb clinician and teacher. He died prematurely, and his absence is keenly felt by his family and his colleagues at both the Children's Hospital in Boston and elsewhere. The third edition was published with the aid of David K. Urion at the Children's Hospital in Boston and was dedicated to Dr. Michael Bresnan. For the fourth edition, we are indebted to Michael E. Cohen and Patricia K. Duffner, of the Children's Hospital of Buffalo. They have taken responsibility for this and future editions, and they completely reorganized the book and updated the content and references to make it even more reader friendly than the previous editions were. We hope that *Pediatric Neurology* continues to meet the need for a readable, pocket-sized, practical reference for pediatric neurologic illness.

Howard L. Weiner, M.D.
Lawrence P. Levitt, M.D.

About the Authors

Michael E. Cohen, M.D., Professor of Neurology and Pediatrics at the State University of New York at Buffalo, was formerly the Chairman of the Department of Neurology at the University at Buffalo. He is now an attending neurologist at the Children's Hospital of Buffalo and the Clinical Director of Neurology Services for the Kaleida Health System. He attended the University at Buffalo School of Medicine & Biological Sciences. He received his neurologic training at the University Hospitals of Cleveland in Cleveland, Ohio and his child neurology training at Boston Children's Hospital. His main interests are in the areas of clinical pediatric neurology and central nervous system tumors of childhood.

Patricia K. Duffner, M.D., Professor of Neurology and Pediatrics at the State University of New York at Buffalo, is presently an attending physician at the Children's Hospital of Buffalo. A graduate of the University of Rochester, she then received her medical training at the State University of New York at Buffalo. She is a frequent lecturer for the American Academy of Pediatrics and the former President of the Section of Neurology of the American Academy of Pediatrics. Her main interests are clinical child neurology and central nervous system neoplasms of childhood, as well as their long-term treatment effects.

About the Series Creators

Howard L. Weiner, M.D., Physician in Medicine (Neurology) at the Brigham and Women's Hospital, is the Robert L. Kroc Professor of Neurology at Harvard Medical School. He graduated from Dartmouth College and then attended the University of Colorado Medical School; he interned at Chaim Sheba Hospital, Tel Hashomer, Israel, and served as a medical resident at the Beth Israel Hospital, Boston. He received his neurology training at the Harvard teaching hospitals of the Longwood Area Neurology Program. Dr. Weiner is the Director of the Partners Multiple Sclerosis program at the Brigham and Women's and Massachusetts General Hospitals and Codirector of the Center for Neurologic Diseases at the Brigham and Women's Hospital.

Lawrence P. Levitt, M.D., Senior Consultant in Neurology at Lehigh Valley Hospital in Allentown, Pennsylvania, is a Professor of Clinical Neurology at Pennsylvania State University College of Medicine. A graduate of Queens College, he attended Cornell Medical College as a Jonas Salk Scholar. Dr. Levitt completed his internship and his first year of residency at Bellevue Hospital, and he then spent 2 years in the Public Health Service at the Encephalitis Research Center in Tampa, Florida. He did his neurology training at the Harvard teaching hospitals of the Longwood Area Neurology Program.

Preface

This manual is designed to guide house officers in recognizing and treating pediatric neurologic disease. It is not intended to be encyclopedic, but it should instead serve as a point of departure for many of the problems encountered by residents in child neurology, pediatrics, adult neurology, and child psychiatry; students; and others interested in child neurology. This manual is the outgrowth of a similar adult manual written for the House Officer Series. The favorable response to the adult manual and the demand of our colleagues for a comparable title covering pediatric neurology have been the impetus behind this book. In keeping with the adult manual, we tried to retain a problem-oriented approach wherever possible, and we hope that the manual fills the need for a readable, pocket-sized, practical reference to the neurologic problems of pediatric patients.

Our desire with regard to this manual is that it will not only excite the intellect of those interested in the nervous system in children but will also provide a point of departure for further inquiry. Interested readers are directed to review articles and major textbooks of child neurology. Resources can be found in the Suggested Reading at the end of each chapter.

Michael E. Cohen, M.D.
Patricia K. Duffner, M.D.

Acknowledgments

We are most grateful to Dr. Levitt for asking us to write this edition of *Pediatric Neurology,* part of the House Officer Series.

We also acknowledge the secretarial support of Linda Amaro, who worked above and beyond the call of duty in helping us complete this text.

Contents

Foreword vi
About the Authors vii
About the Series Creators viii
Preface ix
Acknowledgments xi

1. GROWTH AND DEVELOPMENT 1
In order to assess neurologic problems in childhood fully, a strong knowledge of growth and development is important. This chapter reviews the reflexes and disappearing signs in the newborn and provides an outline of the key developmental milestones in childhood. It serves as a point of departure in helping the examiner differentiate normal from abnormal.

2. NEUROANATOMY 6
This chapter outlines key anatomic features and provides a frame of reference for establishing localization in the nervous system. Anatomic localization is pivotal in understanding multiple causes of neurologic dysfunction. A thorough grounding in anatomy allows the examiner to make the appropriate diagnosis.

3. NEUROLOGIC HISTORY 24
Some have said that 90% of diagnosis is history. This chapter outlines the salient features of neurologic history that should be obtained regarding the intrauterine, perinatal, and neonatal periods.

4. NEUROLOGIC EXAMINATION 27
This chapter describes the neurologic examination in detail, with particular emphasis on the assessment of the preterm, as well as the term, infant. The neurologic examination is predicated on the observation that

the nervous system of the infant from term until early childhood is a dynamic and changing process. Standard neurologic examination is described in some detail.

5. FLOPPY INFANT 44
This chapter provides a frame of reference for evaluating the floppy infant. The causes of the floppy infant syndrome—ranging from diseases of the cerebral cortex to those of the peripheral nervous system—are discussed in detail. An algorithm for evaluating the child who presents with hypotonia in the first several months of life is included.

6. BACK PAIN 56
This chapter discusses both chronic and acute causes of back pain. Both anatomic defects and specific syndromes are discussed. The chapter focuses on back pain as a presenting symptom, but it includes problems not only of the back but also of the spine, roots, and peripheral nerves. This chapter complements the chapter on spinal cord disease. Both compressive disease and noncompressive spinal cord injuries are described.

7. SPINAL CORD DISEASE 61
This chapter discusses the characteristic signs and symptoms of acute and chronic diseases of the spinal cord. Etiologies of both compressive and noncompressive diseases of the spinal cord are presented.

8. NEUROPATHIES 66
This chapter describes the various genetic and nongenetic causes of diseases affecting the peripheral nervous system in childhood. Birth-related injuries, chronic and acute diseases of the peripheral nervous system, compressive neuropathies, and infectious and genetic etiologies primarily affecting the peripheral nerves are outlined. A discussion of the most common illnesses affecting the peripheral nerves and their clinical significance is presented.

9. MUSCLE DISEASES 78
Muscle disease is a common problem in childhood. The various congenital myopathies and dystrophies are described in some detail. An attempt is made to differentiate myopathies from dystrophies. Dermatomyositis is presented as an example of an inflammatory myopathy.

10. MYASTHENIA GRAVIS 89
The various myasthenia gravis syndromes are described in this chapter. The syndromes of neonatal myasthenia, congenital myasthenia, and classical myasthenia are differentiated. Appropriate diagnosis and treatment are discussed.

11. CEREBRAL PALSY 93
Cerebral palsy is classically described as a static, nonprogressive disorder of the central nervous system arising from prenatal or perinatal damage, with or without associated cognitive abnormalities. The various causes and presentations of cerebral palsy are outlined. The text prepares the reader to be readily able to differentiate the various forms of cerebral palsy, provides their etiologies, and suggests treatments.

12. HEMIPARESIS AND STROKE 100
Hemiparesis—weakness of one side of the body—results from lesions of the cortex, subcortex, diencephalon, midbrain, or brainstem. The vascular and nonvascular causes of hemiparesis and their sites of localization are discussed.

13. DEVELOPMENTAL DISABILITIES 113
Developmental disabilities and mental retardation affect up to 5% of children. This chapter outlines an approach to the static and nonprogressive forms of developmental disabilities seen in childhood. Specific reference is made to developmental language disorders, and a description of the classic mental retardation syndromes is provided.

14. PROGRESSIVE DEGENERATIVE DISEASE 120
Dementia is defined as regression from previous levels of function. This is differentiated from failure to achieve or the slow acquisition of developmental milestones. While these latter conditions imply a static condition, dementia suggests a progressive disorder. Many of these abnormalities present prior to 2 years of age. However, some have their onset later on in childhood. This chapter describes degenerative diseases, including those beginning both before and after the age of 2 years.

15. NEUROCUTANEOUS SYNDROMES 130
Neurocutaneous syndromes are disorders that affect both the skin and the central nervous system. The most common neurocutaneous disorders in childhood are discussed in this chapter, which focuses on the clinical presentation, genetics, clinical course, and treatment of these disorders.

16. INFECTIOUS DISEASE 144
This chapter outlines infections affecting the central nervous system. It differentiates meningitis from encephalitis and brain abscess. Bacterial, viral, and other infectious etiologies are discussed, and the approach to diagnosis and therapy is outlined.

17. SEIZURES 155
The various seizure syndromes seen in childhood are outlined in this chapter. Seizure disorders presenting at different times of life are discussed in detail. The typical electroencephalographic features of the various seizure syndromes, as well as an approach to their evaluation and treatment, are presented.

18. FEBRILE SEIZURES 168
The current consensus on the approach to simple febrile seizures in childhood is presented. The American Academy of Pediatrics Practice Parameters are discussed in detail, including the evaluation of the child with a first simple febrile seizure and recommendations

regarding long-term anticonvulsant therapy. Complex febrile seizures are also discussed.

19. NEONATAL SEIZURES 173
Neonatal seizures are seizures occurring specifically in the neonatal period. They present differently from seizures manifesting at other times of life. Unlike seizures beyond the neonatal period, for the most part, the seizures encountered at this time have an etiology. The types of seizures, their clinical presentation, and the appropriate treatment are discussed.

20. NONEPILEPTIC PAROXYSMAL EVENTS 177
Many syndromes in childhood may mimic seizures, even though they are nonepileptic in nature. These include vasovagal syncope, syncope of cardiac origin, the pallid and the cyanotic forms of breath-holding that are seen in infancy, and pseudo seizures. Each of these is described in some detail.

21. SLEEP DISORDERS 181
This chapter describes the most common sleep disorders—narcolepsy, sleep apnea, and central alveolar hypoventilation—as well as the parasomnias, including night tremors, restless legs, sleepwalking, nightmares, and enuresis.

22. COMPLICATIONS OF ANTIEPILEPTIC DRUGS 186
Each year, more antiepileptic drugs are available for the treatment of seizures. A template for the ideal antiepileptic drug is described. The various antiepileptics currently in use are fitted into this template. The newer anticonvulsants and their side effects are presented.

23. GENETICS 197
Increasingly, genetic syndromes of the nervous system are being identified and codified. The various forms of mendelian and mitochondrial inheritance are discussed. An approach to the evaluation of the various genetic problems is presented.

consciousness. Particular attention is paid to head trauma, increased intracranial pressure, and herniation syndromes.

30. GAIT 246
Disorders of gait are quite common in childhood. They can involve any part of the neural axis. This chapter provides an anatomic framework for evaluating these problems.

31. CEREBELLAR ATAXIA 250
The cerebellum is a common shock organ in the child's nervous system. Cerebellar disease can present in both an acute and a chronic fashion. This chapter outlines the evaluation of the patient who presents with a cerebellar syndrome.

32. MOVEMENT DISORDERS 257
Movement disorders are complex disorders of motion that defy easy editorial description; they must be visualized to be appreciated. Most of these are choreic or athetotic in nature. They may be either intermittent or paroxysmal. This chapter discusses those movement abnormalities presenting as chorea, athetosis, and dystonias.

33. OTHER MOVEMENT DISORDERS: MYOCLONUS, TICS, AND TREMORS 264
In addition to chorea or athetosis, other movement disorders of childhood require definition and classification. These include myoclonus, tics, and tremors. This chapter provides the differential diagnosis for and the treatment of these disorders.

34. PERVASIVE DEVELOPMENTAL DISORDERS 268
Disorders of behavior and impulse control are major problems in childhood. This chapter discusses the entire spectrum of pervasive development disorders and offers a perspective on their diagnosis, identification, and treatment.

35. ATTENTION DEFICIT HYPERACTIVITY DISORDER 274
Attention deficit hyperactivity disorders may affect more than 15% of children. The syndrome itself is largely descriptive as its biologic parameters are limited. While keeping in mind that physicians should rely on their knowledge of the syndrome and of family dynamics to make the diagnosis, the chapter does provide an approach to diagnosis and treatment.

36. VERTIGO 277
The assessment of the child with vertigo can be complex; it includes a careful history and neurologic examination. This chapter reviews the differential diagnosis of acute and chronic vertigo, both with and without hearing loss, and distinguishes vertigo from light-headedness.

37. LUMBAR PUNCTURE AND CEREBROSPINAL FLUID EXAMINATION 283
This chapter outlines methods for, contraindications to, and complications of lumbar puncture. Interpretation of cerebrospinal fluid abnormalities and discussion of disorders that affect the cerebrospinal fluid are presented in outline form.

APPENDICES

I. KEY DEVELOPMENTAL MILESTONES 289

II. NEWBORN MATURITY RATING AND CLASSIFICATION 293

III. HEAD CIRCUMFERENCE FOR AGE PERCENTILES 300

IV. AGE OF COPYING FIGURES 303

V. APGAR SCORE 305

VI. GLASGOW COMA SCALE 306

Chapter 1

Growth and Development

All those who care for children should have a working knowledge of growth and development, specifically in assessing the child under 2 years of age. The first year of life is a period in which the child rapidly acquires new skills. Developmental milestones are rapidly attained during the first year of life. At birth, the child primarily sleeps and feeds. However, by the end of the first year, the child is usually walking independently and is saying a few words. By the end of the second year, the child is fully ambulatory; he or she has developed fine motor skills, climbs stairs, has a well-established hand preference, begins to speak in sentences; and, furthermore, he or she is well on the road to toilet training. Two-year-old children are highly social, they know their parents and siblings, they interact with the environment, and they tend to have significant stranger anxiety (see Appendix I: Key Developmental Milestones).

The average head circumference of the newborn child is between 34 and 35.5 cm. The head circumference provides the examiner with an idea of the child's brain volume and mass. Either a large head or a small head is abnormal, and the presence of either one should initiate appropriate investigative measures. As a general rule, during the first 3 months of life, the child's head will grow at the rate of 2 cm a month. Over the next 3 months, head growth is approximately 1 cm a month and then, over the next 6 months, is approximately 0.5 cm a month. By the end of the first year of life, the child's head circumference will have grown somewhere between 9 and 12 cm. Remember, three-fourths of the individual's head growth will occur within the first several years of life (see

Appendix II: Newborn Maturity Rating and Classification and Appendix III: Head Circumference for Age Percentiles).

REFLEXES AND DISAPPEARING SIGNS

Moro Reflex

The Moro reflex is a startle reaction that consists of abduction of the arms, extension of the legs, and flexion of the hips. It is present in all normal, full-term children. The Moro reflex indicates symmetry of the nervous system and the intactness of the spinal cord and lower brainstem. At 4 to 5 months of age, the Moro reflex is usually lost.

Tonic Neck Reflex

A tonic neck reflex is obtained when the head is turned from one side to the other with the infant in the supine position. This results in the extension of the arm while lying on the side with flexion of the contralateral arm, or the so-called fencing position. The age at which the tonic neck reflex is first elicited has not been universally recognized. It is generally appreciated at 2 to 3 weeks of age, and it disappears well into the first year. The tonic neck reflex fatigues early, and it is never obligate. When the infant is turned to one side, the child will break that position after a few seconds. The persistence of an obligate tonic reflex is associated with asymmetric central nervous system development, and it may predict the development of choreoathetotic cerebral palsy.

Crossed Adductor Reflex and Other Pyramidal Signs

The crossed adductor reflex consists of contraction of both hip adductors when either knee jerk is elicited. This usually disappears by 7 to 8 months. Persistence beyond this time is considered an early sign of pyramidal tract dysfunction. Ankle clonus may be found in the newborn; this generally disappears by 2 to 3 months of age. It should never be sustained, however. A tentative Babinski reflex is considered normal either until 1 year of age or when the child begins to bear weight. Most authors consider a Babinski sign inconsequential unless the child is either bearing weight or walking, his or her reflexes are abnormal, or the Babinski is asymmetric. With these considerations in mind, the Babinski then points to signs of pyramidal tract dysfunction.

Grasp Reflex

Palmer grasping occurs at birth and disappears by 4 to 5 months of age; it is replaced by voluntary and inferior pincer grasping. The acquisition of a normal pincer grasp is seen between 9 and 15 months of age. This is a sure sign that cortical motor development is on target. Even at birth, a child's hands will be open approximately 50% of the time. If the hands are not fully opened by 3 months of age as the child begins to explore the environment, a suspicion of pyramidal dysfunction should be raised.

Placing and Stepping

Placing and stepping occur at birth and may persist until the child bears weight. These reflexes are elicited by stroking the dorsal surface of the foot. After stimulation, the child will lift his or her foot over a tabletop or chair. This is a newborn reflex that will disappear with increasing age.

Parachute Reflex

The parachute reflex occurs when a youngster is held in a horizontal position and is then thrust downward. This reflex consists of arm extension to break the fall; it is a normal postural supporting reaction. It is well developed by 6 to 7 months of age. The parachute reflex is a good sign of upper extremity motor development. If it is asymmetric, it may be an early sign of pyramidal disease.

Landau Response

Holding the child in a horizontal position is a test of head control and motor function. At 4 months of age, the infant will hold the head horizontally parallel to the ground and will begin to arch his or her back. The legs tend to be flexor in ventral suspension.

Hand Use

An open hand is a good sign of normal motor cortical development. An infant is able to reach and grasp with his or her whole hand by 4 to 5 months of age. Transferring objects from one hand to the other begins at 7 to 8 months of age. Strong hand preference is usually abnormal before 1 year of age; however, ambidexterity is not specifically abnormal.

Babinski Reflex

This reflex is present at birth and is normal until the child bears weight. This reflex may persist through the first year of life.

GENERAL ASSESSMENT

The two most reliable signs that an infant is developing normal intelligence are the early onset of pincer grasp and/or the early acquisition of language. The child develops a normal pincer grasp by 9 to 15 months of age. This finding alone is assurance that the child's nervous system is intact. Similarly, acquisition of speech by 1 year of age suggests a normal intelligence. Speech, however, may be delayed in many normal children until 3 or even 4 years of age.

A useful tool to assess developmental milestones is the Denver Developmental Test. This outlines in percentage form the gross motor skills, fine motor skills, language, and personal and social milestones chronicled over a multiple year period. The Denver Developmental Test is not a test of intellectual function. Accurate intellectual function can be best obtained by formal psychometric examinations after 4 to 5 years of age. Cognitive tests such as the Bailey Scale for Infants, although they do provide some suggestion of normal development, correlate poorly with the standardized intellectual tests used in children 4 to 5 years of age and older. Appendix IV indicates the approximate age at which children can copy various figures.

Key developmental milestones are as follows:

1. Smiling spontaneously between 1 to 3 months.
2. Smiling responsively at 6 to 8 weeks.
3. Reaching at 4 to 6 months.
4. Following with the eyes through 180 degrees at 12 to 16 weeks.
5. Drinking from a cup at 9 to 15 months.
6. Developing a pincer grasp at 9 to 15 months.
7. Initiating and imitating sounds and babbling at 6 months.
8. Combining words at 15 to 18 months.
9. Learning colors within the second year of life.
10. Bearing weight at 2 to 6 months of age.
11. Pulling to sit with no head lag at 4 to 6 months.
12. Sitting without support at 7 to 10 months.

13. Standing unsupported at 9 to 11 months.
14. Walking without assistance at 9 to 18 months.

In the older child, information concerning cognition can be obtained from the school, teacher questionnaire evaluations, or group tests such as the Otis-Lennon. These tests are given to children throughout their school years, and they are useful for comparison among specific age groups. School reports will not only supply information concerning academic skills, but they will also reveal multiple aspects of behavior motivation, attention, and attendance. A professional psychologist can best assess specific tests of intellect.

Suggested Reading

Finberg L, Kleinman RE, eds. *Saunders manual of pediatric practice,* 2nd ed. Philadelphia: W. B. Saunders, 2002.

Menkes JH, Sarnat HB, eds. *Child neurology,* 6th ed. Philadelphia: Lippincott Williams & Wilkins, 2000.

Swaiman KF, Ashwal S. *Pediatric neurology: principles and practice.* St Louis: Mosby, 1999.

Chapter 2

Neuroanatomy

LOCALIZATION

As in adult neurology, attempts to localize a lesion are the prelude to accurate diagnosis and treatment. Additionally, in the child, the question of whether the nervous system has matured appropriately for the child's age must be answered. Hence, for the pediatric neurologist, a comprehensive knowledge of neuroanatomy, neurophysiology, growth, and development is imperative. The ability to localize a lesion requires a knowledge of both the horizontal and the vertical organization of the nervous system. Consider localization in a cephalocaudal manner (i.e., from top to bottom). For the most part, intellectual function resides in the cortex. However, children with developmental or congenital absence of tissue may have normal to near normal intellect. This is an example of the plasticity of the nervous system of children, unlike that of adults. Increasingly as disease becomes more caudal, the motor and sensory systems are equally involved. Midline involvement of the nervous system primarily involving the diencephalon and mesencephalon will have an impact on vital functions, such as breathing, waking, sleeping, eating, and swallowing. Unlike respiratory function, cardiac status, for the most part, is independent of nervous system control. Involvement of the cortical white matter results in contralateral motor and sensory loss.

Periventricular lesions may cause spastic diplegia, wherein the legs are involved with relative sparing of the arms. This occurs because leg fibers, which descend from the cortex through the centrum semiovale, the internal capsule, and the cerebral peduncles, and subsequently pass into the brainstem and spinal cord, are more medially located than are the arm fibers. As a result, periventricular lesions involve the more medially located leg fibers with sparing of the more lateral arm fibers. Lesions of the internal capsule tend to involve the face, arm, and leg uniformly, whereas lesions of the subcortex are more likely to be facial, brachial, or crural in presentation.

In the brainstem, systems subserving the cerebellum, cortex, and cranial nerves are located in a small anatomic space. Hence, a triad of long tract signs, cerebellar signs, and cranial neuropathies characterizes brainstem lesions. Spinal cord lesions, on the other hand, depending on their level, affect the arm, thorax, or lower extremities. In the spinal cord, the findings of pain and temperature loss contralateral to proprioception, light touch, and long tract signs suggest a hemisection of the cord. Involvement of a root entry zone with the loss of reflexes at the level of the lesion and hyperreflexia and long tract signs below the lesion also suggest a spinal cord localization. A sensory level localizes the lesion to the spinal cord. Involvement of the bowel and bladder localizes the lesion to the conus medullaris or epiconus, whereas involvement in the distribution of a peripheral nerve, whether motor, sensory, or in combination, limits the location to either a root or peripheral nerve.

Anatomic orientation is not just an intellectual exercise. Knowledge of location often leads to the appropriate diagnosis and subsequent treatment. A useful example is the evaluation of the child with hypotonia. Hypotonia may be a nonspecific sign, and it can relate to dysfunction at any point in the neuraxis from the cerebral cortex through the cerebellum, spinal cord, nerve roots, and peripheral nerves. In fact, the appropriate assessment of the floppy infant depends on the ability to unravel this complex presentation. Paraparesis, spastic diplegia, monoplegias, and foot drop may all have variable presentations within the neuraxis. Ataxia can reflect a cortical, brainstem, cerebellar, or peripheral nervous system disease. Finally, a comprehensive understanding of the nervous system is imperative in sorting out hysterical signs and symptoms, which surprisingly are quite common in childhood. Each of these problems is discussed in detail in further sections.

The nervous system does not exist in isolation. Although this seems self-evident, assessment must result in a determination of whether the primary problem is neurologic or if it lies outside the nervous system. Multiple systemic causes of disease can indirectly affect neurologic function. Some may cause changes in posture and consciousness. Others produce autonomic and behavioral abnormalities or confusional states. After neurologic assessment, a generic category of disease as one of the following should be established: developmental, metabolic, neoplastic, intoxicant, degenerative, endocrine, or vascular.

KEY POINTS IN NEUROANATOMY

The cerebral cortex is comprised of four lobes for each hemisphere, and each lobe has specialized functions (Fig. 2.1)

1. *Frontal* lobes participate in speech (Broca's area for speech is in the dominant hemisphere), movement (the corticospinal tracts originate here), personality, and initiative. Frontal eye fields participate in conjugate eye deviation so that lesions on one side cause the eye to deviate to the ipsilateral side.
2. *Temporal* lobes participate in memory functions and auditory processing. For language, the involvement of the dominant

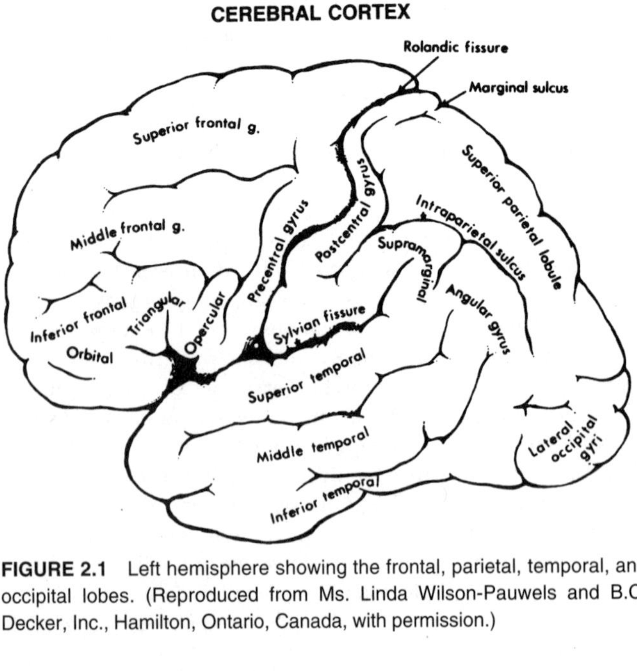

FIGURE 2.1 Left hemisphere showing the frontal, parietal, temporal, and occipital lobes. (Reproduced from Ms. Linda Wilson-Pauwels and B.C. Decker, Inc., Hamilton, Ontario, Canada, with permission.)

hemisphere is seen; for music, usually the nondominant hemisphere is active. A unilateral temporal lesion may cause a contralateral superior quadrantanopsia as a result of the involvement of optic radiations.

3. The *parietal* cortex participates in sensation; thus, the contralateral loss of cortical sensation occurs with lesions (e.g., two point discrimination, identification of objects, or numbers drawn in the hand). A mild hemiparesis may occur with parietal injury; alexia, agraphia, left–right discrimination difficulty, and finger naming difficulty occur with a lesion in the left angular gyrus of the parietal lobe. Nondominant parietal lesions may cause visuospatial difficulty, dressing apraxia, loss of awareness of the left side of the body, and topographic memory loss.
4. The *occipital* lobes participate in vision. Lesions of the occipital lobe cause visual field loss, hallucinosis, or blindness. Altered recognition of objects or faces by sight may also occur.

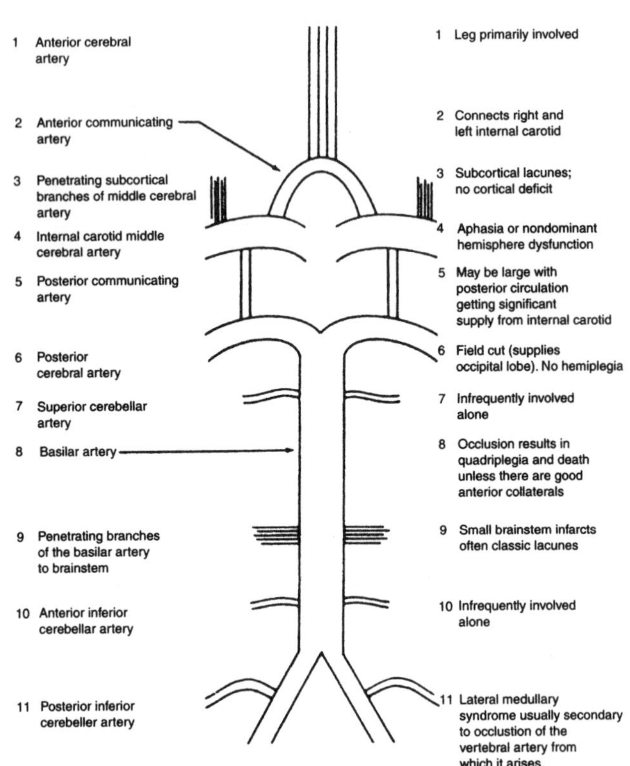

FIGURE 2.2 Cerebral circulation. (From Weiner HL, Levitt LP, Rae-Grant A. *Neurology*, 6th ed. Philadelphia: Lippincott Williams & Wilkins, 1999, with permission.)

The anterior, middle, and posterior cerebral arteries supply, respectively, the anteromesial cortex; the lateral frontal, temporal, and parietal lobes; and the occipital lobes. The superior cerebellar artery supplies the superior aspect of the cerebellum. The basilar artery supplies the upper brainstem, and the vertebral arteries supply the lower brainstem and cerebellum. The anastomotic circle of Willis connects the anterior and posterior circulation through the posterior communicating arteries and the left and right circulations through the anterior communicating artery (Fig. 2.2). The circle of Willis is frequently anatomically incomplete.

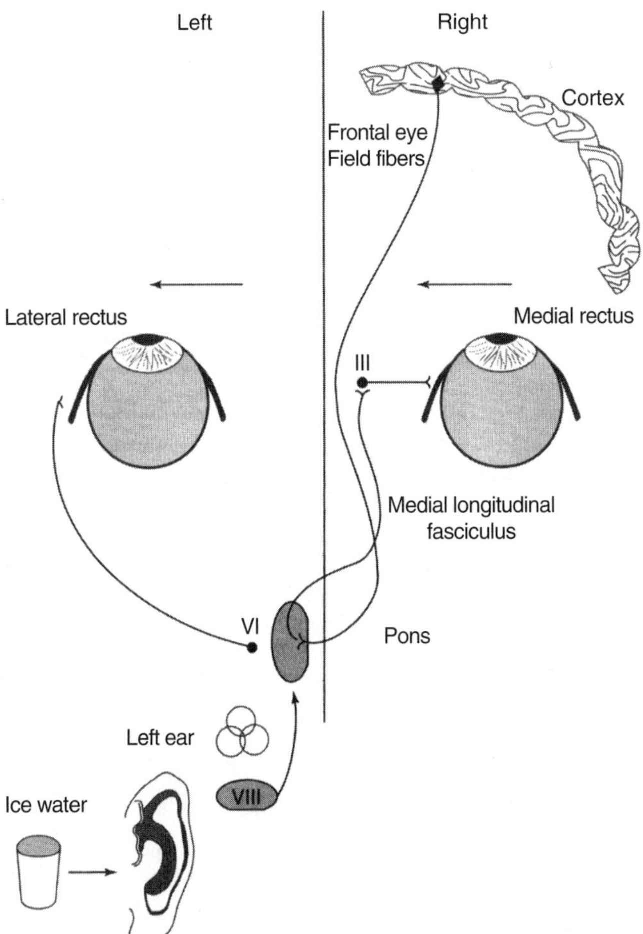

FIGURE 2.3 In the comatose patient with an intact brainstem, ice water in the left ear causes deviation of the eyes to the left. In the awake patient, this deviation is counteracted voluntarily, producing nystagmus to the right. (From Weiner HL, Levitt LP, Rae-Grant A. *Neurology*, 6th ed. Philadelphia: Lippincott Williams & Wilkins, 1999, with permission.)

The frontal eye fields exert a major influence on horizontal eye movement, with each field being concerned with contralateral eye deviation. Thus, the right field causes the eyes to move to the left. (The fibers cross in the pons and connect there to the extraocular muscles via the medial longitudinal fasciculus.) Both fields are constantly active, striking a balance; thus, when one is more or less active than the other, horizontal eye deviation results (Fig. 2.3).

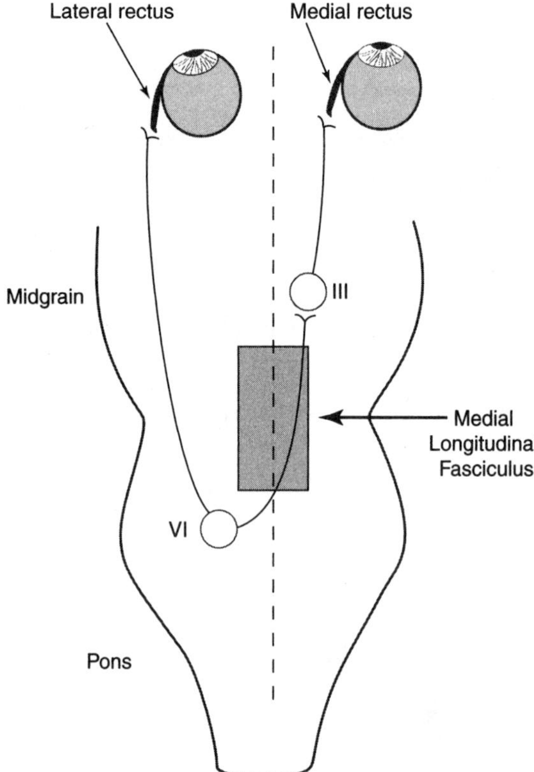

FIGURE 2.4 Horizontal eye movements. (From Weiner HL, Levitt LP, Rae-Grant A. *Neurology*, 6th ed. Philadelphia: Lippincott Williams & Wilkins, 1999, with permission.)

Horizontal eye movements are subserved by the medial (third nerve) and lateral (sixth nerve) rectus muscles (Fig. 2.4). Inputs from the cortex and eighth nerve nuclei affect the parapontine reticular formation, which drives the sixth nerve nucleus. This stimulates the ipsilateral lateral rectus and the contralateral medial rectus, connecting with the latter through the medial longitudinal fasciculus. A lesion in the sixth nerve nucleus causes a paralysis of the ipsilateral gaze (the individual cannot bring the eyes to the injured side because of weakness in the ipsilateral lateral rectus.

A *destructive lesion* in the hemisphere or subcortex causes the eyes to deviate toward the same side as the lesion. Thus, with a right-sided lesion, the eyes are deviated to the right. An *excitatory lesion* at the cortical level (e.g., a seizure) causes the eyes to deviate to the contralateral side. A *destructive lesion* in the pons causes the eyes to deviate to the side opposite the damage. Thus, with a left-sided lesion, eyes deviate to the right. Eye deviation secondary to hemisphere lesions, but not to brainstem lesions, may be overcome by brainstem reflexes (e.g., the doll's eye maneuver) (Fig. 2.4).

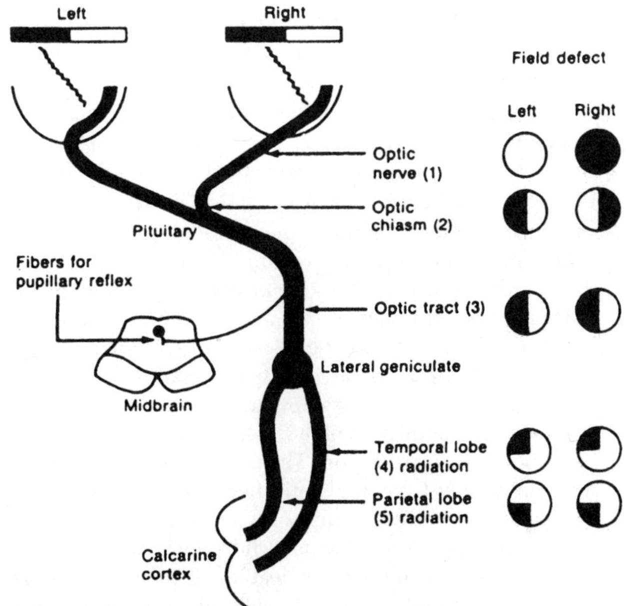

FIGURE 2.5 Visual pathways. (From Weiner HL, Levitt LP, Rae-Grant A. *Neurology*, 6th ed. Philadelphia: Lippincott Williams & Wilkins, 1999, with permission.)

1. *Blindness in one eye* represents retinal or ipsilateral optic nerve dysfunction (Fig. 2.5). The optic nerve is frequently involved

in multiple sclerosis (optic neuritis), producing unilateral blindness; it may also be involved by tumor (optic glioma) or it may undergo atrophy secondary to prolonged increased intracranial pressure. Vascular processes, such as giant cell arteritis and amaurosis fugax, may also affect the optic nerve.

2. *Bitemporal hemianopsia* is classically found in the pituitary tumors secondary to pressure on the optic chiasm. Nonhomonymous field defects usually imply lesions near the chiasm. Remember, concentric tunnel vision may be seen in hysterical blindness.
3. *Homonymous hemianopsia* implies a lesion posterior to the chiasm. It may involve the optic tract or optic radiations emanating from the lateral geniculate body (or the lateral geniculate itself). The closer a lesion is to the lateral geniculate, the smaller it can be while still producing a homonymous hemianopsia. Occlusions of the posterior cerebral artery usually produce a homonymous hemianopsia with sparing of the macula.
4. The *optic radiations* fan out from the lateral geniculate and travel in the temporal and parietal lobes before reaching their destination in the occipital lobe. Lesions in the temporal lobe may give a homonymous superior field defect if the optic radiations are affected. Similarly, a lesion in the parietal lobe may show an inferior homonymous field defect.
5. When one realizes the large territory needed for *intact visual fields,* the reason that checking visual fields is a mandatory part of every neurologic examination becomes apparent.
6. *Pupillary response* must also be assessed. The pupil depends on input from both the parasympathetic nervous system via the third cranial nerves and sympathetic inputs. Lesions of the third nerve cause dilation of the third nerve; lesions of the sympathetics cause constriction. The pupillary light reflex has an afferent supply from the optic nerve, through the lateral geniculate nucleus of the thalamus, to the midbrain pretectal area to the third nerve. Horner syndrome is caused by a sympathetic disorder of the fibers leading to the pupil and face. Miosis (small pupil), ptosis (partial), and anhidrosis (caused by sweat gland innervation to the face on the same side) are seen in combination. The sympathetics travel from the hypothalamus through the brainstem, the spinal cord to T-1 or T-2, out the roots to near the apex of the lung, up the carotid sheath, and in with the ophthalmic artery.

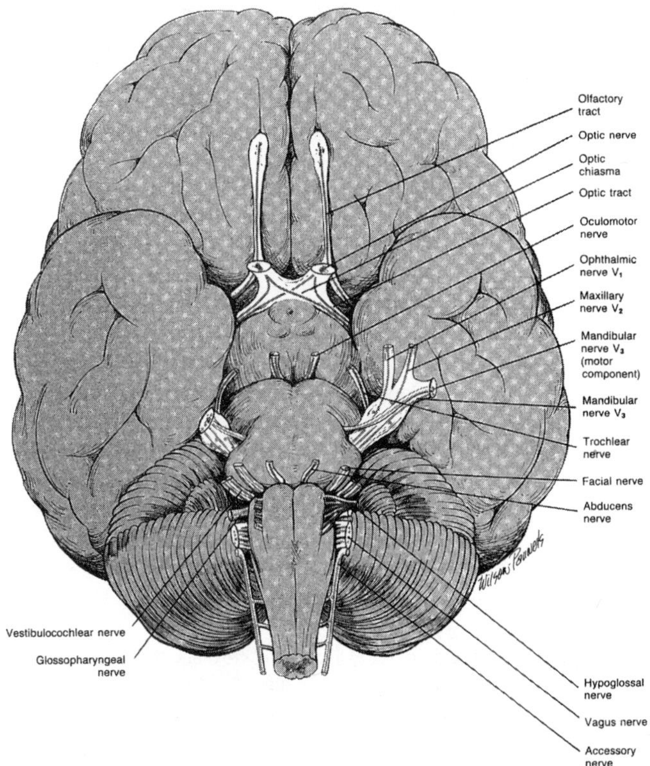

FIGURE 2.6 Base of the brain. (From Ms. Linda Wilson-Pauwels and B.C. Decker, Inc., Hamilton, Ontario, Canada, with permission.)

Remember, the first and second cranial nerves lie outside the brainstem. The third and fourth are in the midbrain, the fifth through eighth are in the pons, and the ninth through twelfth are in the medulla (Figs. 2.6 to 2.10)

I—olfactory, in the mesial cortex; rhinencephalon. Smell.

II—optic nerve, enters at the lateral geniculate body. Visual function.

III—oculomotor nerve, midbrain. Innervates the medial, superior, and inferior rectus; the inferior oblique; the lid elevator; and the pupil.

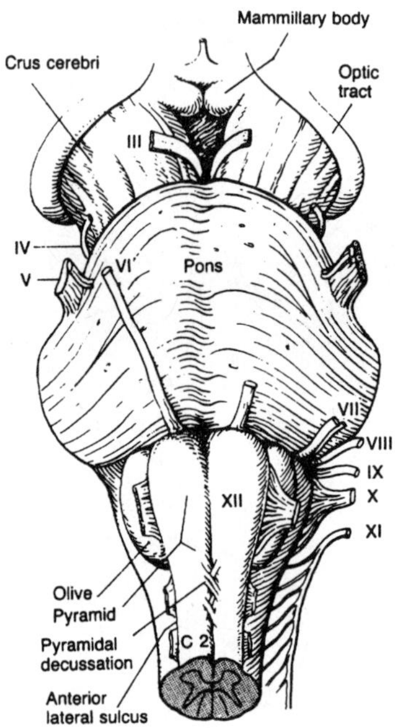

FIGURE 2.7 The cranial nerves at the base of the brain. (From Duus P. *Topical diagnosis in neurology*. New York: Thieme, 1983, with permission.)

IV—trochlear nerve, midbrain. Innervates the superior oblique. Brings the eye down and in.
V—trigeminal, pons (and medulla). Supplies the muscles of mastication, facial sensation, corneal reflex.
VI—abducens, pons. Supplies the lateral rectus, brings the eye outward.
VII—facial. Supplies facial movements, tearing, and salivation.
VIII—auditory. Supplies hearing and vestibular function.
IX—glossopharyngeal. Supplies palatal sensation.
X—vagus. Supplies muscles of swallowing, autonomic parasympathetics to internal organs.
XI—spinal accessory nerve. Supplies sternocleidomastoid and trapezius muscles.
XII—hypoglossal. Supplies muscles of the tongue.

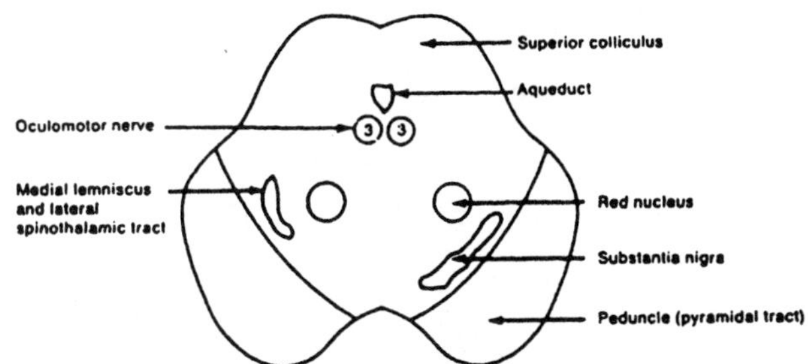

FIGURE 2.8 Midbrain (cranial nerves 3 to 4). (From Weiner HL, Levitt LP, Rae-Grant A. *Neurology*, 6th ed. Philadelphia: Lippincott Williams & Wilkins, 1999, with permission.)

Midbrain

The most prominent disturbance in the midbrain (Fig. 2.8) generally involves the third nerve nucleus or exiting fibers, producing a dilated pupil and ophthalmoplegia. Lesions affecting the area of the midbrain at the level of the superior colliculus produce difficulty with upward gaze, convergence, and pupillary light reflexes (Parinaud syndrome). A tumor pressing on the superior colliculus may present in this way (e.g., pinealoma).

Lesions of the red nucleus produce contralateral ataxia and tremor (rubral tremor). The substantia nigra is located at this level, and it plays an important role in Parkinson disease. The fourth nerve nucleus is also located in the midbrain at a lower level, and it seldom is involved alone (e.g., because of trauma). Fourth nerve injury causes a head tilt.

Fibers from the optic tract concerned with the pupillary response synapse in the region of third nerve nucleus. Lesions in the midbrain may impair the pupillary reaction to direct light, but they may leave contraction to accommodation intact.

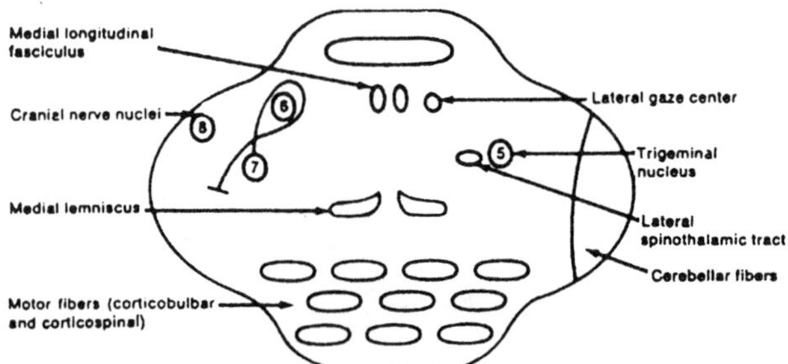

FIGURE 2.9 Pons (cranial nerves 5 to 8). (From Weiner HL, Levitt LP, Rae-Grant A. *Neurology*, 6th ed. Philadelphia: Lippincott Williams & Wilkins, 1999, with permission.)

Pons

The fibers of the seventh (facial) nerve sweep around the sixth nerve (lateral rectus) before exiting from the pons (Fig. 2.9). Thus, a lesion at this level often produces a VI and VII nerve paralysis on the same side.

The basic structure of the pons is as follows. Medial involvement produces motor dysfunction and internuclear ophthalmologic or gaze palsy to the side of the lesion. Lateral involvement causes pain and temperature dysfunction.

Vertical nystagmus is a sign of brainstem dysfunction at the level of the pontomedullary junction or upper midbrain, unless the patient is taking barbiturates.

The *eighth nerve nuclei* include cochlear and vestibular components.

The *trigeminal nerve* exits from the middle of the pons, and, if it is involved at this level, produces face pain and ipsilateral loss of the corneal reflex. In high pontine lesions, pain and sensory loss are contralateral to the lesion in the face and extremities. Below the high pons, pain and temperature senses are lost ipsilaterally in the face and contralaterally in the limbs.

Lesions of the *medial longitudinal fasciculus* (MLF) result in an internuclear ophthalmoplegia. If the right MLF is involved, difficulty with right eye adduction is seen, as well as nystagmus in the abducting left eye when the patient looks to the left.

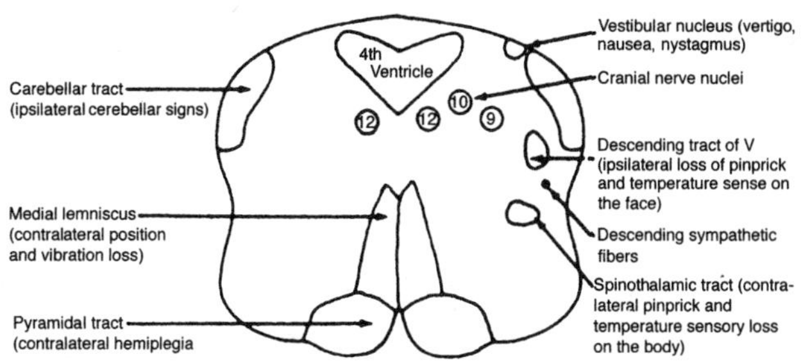

FIGURE 2.10 Medulla (cranial nerves 9 to 12). (From Weiner HL, Levitt LP, Rae-Grant A. *Neurology,* 6th ed. Philadelphia: Lippincott Williams & Wilkins, 1999, with permission.)

Medulla

The most commonly encountered vascular syndrome affecting the medulla (Fig. 2.10) is the *lateral medullary (Wallenberg syndrome),* which defines a major portion of the dysfunction that can be seen with medullary involvement. (Medial structures, such as the pyramids, medial lemniscus, and twelfth nerve nucleus, are unaffected.)

Remember that the *seventh (facial) nerve is not in the medulla;* thus, if facial weakness is present, dysfunction at the level of the pons or above must exist.

When the *descending sympathetic fibers* are involved, an ipsilateral Horner syndrome (ptosis, small pupil, and facial anhidrosis) results.

The cranial nerve nuclei are as follows:

Twelfth (hypoglossal): unilateral involvement of the nucleus causes fasciculations on that side; when the tongue is protruded, it deviates to the side of the lesion.

Tenth (vagus) and *ninth* (glossopharyngeal): these innervate the laryngeal and pharyngeal musculature; dysphagia is prominent when they are involved.

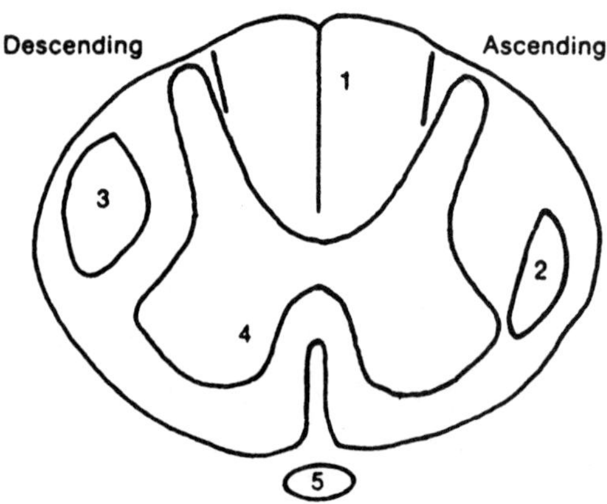

FIGURE 2.11 Spinal cord cross section, showing the dorsal columns (*1*), spinothalamic tracts (*2*), corticospinal tracts (*3*), anterior horns (*4*), and anterior spinal artery (*5*). (From Weiner HL, Levitt LP, Rae-Grant A. *Neurology*, 6th ed. Philadelphia: Lippincott Williams & Wilkins, 1999, with permission.)

Vascular Supply

The *anterior spinal artery* (5) supplies the entire cord except for the dorsal columns. Thus, the anterior spinal artery syndrome produces paralysis and loss of pain and temperature sense; position and vibratory sense are preserved (Fig. 2.11).

CLINICAL CORRELATION

- Subacute combined system disease affects 1 and 3.
- Amyotrophic lateral sclerosis affects 3 and 4.
- Friedreich ataxia affects 1.
- Multiple sclerosis affects 1, 2, and 3 (alone or in combination).
- Infantile spinal muscular atrophy affects 4.
- Brown-Séquard syndrome (hemisection of the cord) produces ipsilateral paralysis, ipsilateral loss of vibration and position sense, and a contralateral loss of sensation to pinprick and temperature.

The *dorsal columns* (1) carry position and vibratory sense; the fibers rise ipsilaterally and cross in the medulla (Table 2.1). These columns are laminated, but the lamination is usually of little clinical importance.

The *lateral spinothalamic tract* (2) carries pain and temperature sensation. These fibers cross on entering the cord; a cord lesion affecting them produces a contralateral loss. They are laminated with sacral fibers, of which most are laterally placed. Thus, an expanding process in the center of the cord gives sacral sparing (i.e., pinprick and temperature sensory loss are least prominent in the sacral area) (Fig. 2.12, A and B).

TABLE 2.1 Crossings in the Nervous System[a]

Pathway	Function	Crosses	Interpretation
Pyramidal tract	Motor	Lower medulla	Lesion below crossing gives ipsilateral signs
Spinothalamic tract	Pain and temperature (body)	On entry to spinal cord	Lesion is always contralateral to pain and temperature loss (except in face)
Spinal tract of fifth (V) nerve	Pain and temperature (face)	Midpons (runs throughout medulla)	If lesion is in medulla or lower pons, ipsilateral loss; above midpons, contralateral loss
Spinal dorsal columns	Position and vibration	Lower medulla	Lesion below crossing give ipsilateral signs
Cerebellar tracts	Coordination of movement	Crosses twice (on entry to cerebellum and in midbrain)	Because of the "double crossing", lesion of cerebellum or cerebellar tracts usually produces signs and symptoms ipsilateral to lesion
Gaze fibers	Coordinate lateral gaze	Midpons	See Fig. 2.3 for interpretation
Cranial nerve fibers	Cranial nerves	Just above cranial nerve nucleus	Lesion is ipsilateral when cranial nerve nuclei are involved

[a]Almost all major pathways in the nervous system cross. Much of the understanding of neuroanatomy relates to knowing where these tracts cross and thus at which level the nervous system is involved.

Modified from Weiner HL, Levitt LP, Rae-Grant A. *Neurology*, 6th ed. Philadelphia: Lippincott Williams & Wilkins, 1999, with permission.

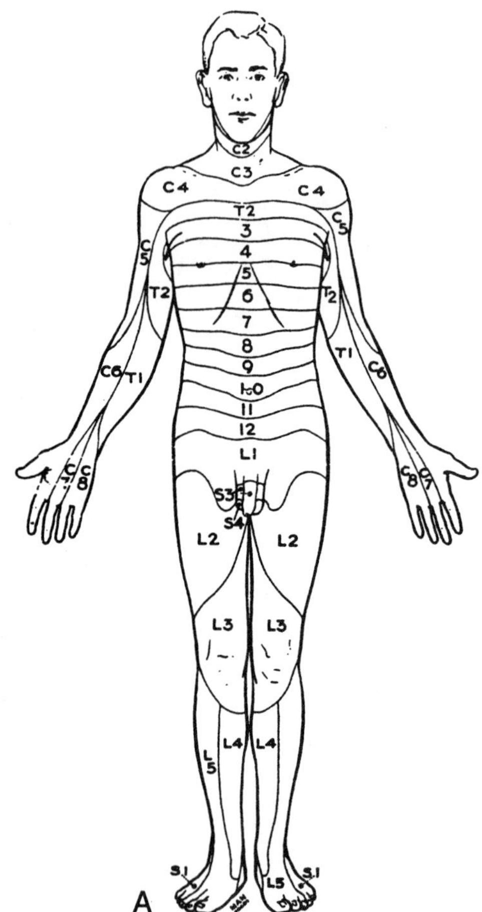

FIGURE 2.12 Dermatome sensory chart. **A:** The dermatomes from the anterior view. (*Continued*)

DESCENDING TRACTS

The *lateral corticospinal tract* (3) carries motor fibers that synapse at the anterior horn cells. The fibers have already crossed in the medulla. A lesion or pressure on the corticospinal tract causes weakness, spasticity, hyperreflexia, and up-going toes.

The *anterior horn cells* (4) are lower motor neurons. A lesion here produces weakness, muscle wasting, fasciculations, and the loss of reflexes and tone.

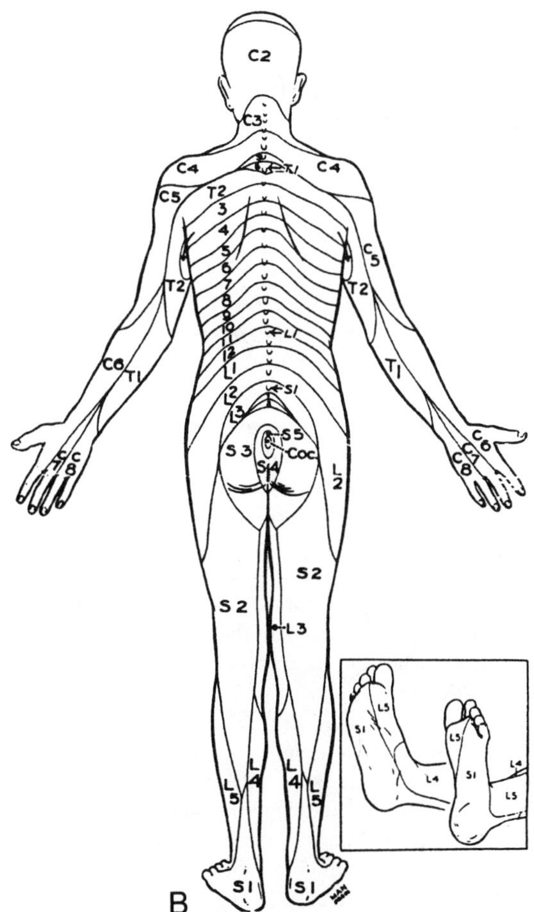

FIGURE 2.12 (*Continued*) **B:** The dermatomes from the posterior view. (From Keegan JJ, Garrett FD. The segmental distribution of the cutaneous nerves in the limbs of man. *Anat Rec* 1948;102:409, with permission.)

Suggested Reading

Menkes JH, Sarnat HB, eds. *Child neurology,* 6th ed. Philadelphia: Lippincott Williams & Wilkins, 2000.

Swaiman KF, Ashwal S. *Pediatric neurology: principles and practice.* St. Louis: Mosby, 1999.

Chapter 3

Neurologic History

Axiomatic in establishing a correct neurologic diagnosis is the ability to obtain an accurate and precise history. History frames the diagnostic possibilities, creates differential diagnoses, anticipates neurologic abnormalities, and establishes a possible familial origin to the complaint. The presenting complaint should be placed in one of several generic diagnostic categories (e.g., developmental, genetic, infectious, intoxicant, metabolic, neoplastic, traumatic, or vascular). Each of these categories may have multiple subsets that should be explored, where appropriate, as the history unfolds.

Ninety-five percent of correct diagnoses come from history and only 5% from the examination. A parent is invariably a better observer of the child than is the physician. The interpretation of symptoms is the obligation of the physician, but the chronicling of historical details by a parent, no matter how imprecise, is usually correct. The maxim remains that the historical record is best obtained from the parent, a caretaker, or the child. After obtaining a history from a parent, reviewing the details with the child, independent of age, is prudent with recognition that even a 3 year old may add some clarification to the presenting complaint. Details of the history should frame the chief complaint. Obtaining a good history requires skill, perseverance, and patience.

Determining whether the process is chronic, acute, static, progressive, degenerative, focal, or generalized is important. Skilled inquiry can assess whether the process under consideration was initiated in the intrauterine, perinatal, or neonatal period. An intrauterine etiology is more common in the very young (under

18 years) or older (over 35 years) mothers. Was the mother ill during the pregnancy, especially during the first trimester? A list of all genetic illnesses in both the mother and father should be obtained. Ultrasonography, increased α-fetal protein, and/or abnormal amniocentesis or chorionic villus biopsy may establish an intrauterine pathology.

Abnormal presentation at birth suggests intrauterine complications, rather than problems at the time of delivery; for example, a breech or transverse lie presentation suggests difficulty in the maternal environment. Small birth weight for gestational age implies problems with maternal–fetal interaction. Clues that suggest intrauterine distress, rather than a neonatal etiology, are meconium staining, premature rupture of membranes, or alterations in heart rate.

Poor Apgar scores (see Appendix V), the need for excessive suctioning at the time of delivery, whether the child was on a ventilator, or a seizure in the first 24 hours of life suggests difficulty in the neonatal period. Failure to suck, failure to thrive in the first week of life, and the onset of seizures after 48 hours suggests an etiology other than a hypoxic–ischemic one. At a minimum, the record should include pregnancy data, birth weight, head circumference, gestational age, and Apgar scores. A record of medications taken by the mother with a description of any illness contracted during the pregnancy should be obtained. Abnormalities in labor and delivery and whether the child was jaundiced, meconium stained, or cyanotic and if he or she had seizures at birth should be documented. The length of time that the child stayed in the hospital should also be recorded.

The historical record should include whether or not a loss of previously obtained milestones has occurred or if the milestones were ever reached. Information should be obtained regarding motor, language, and adaptive behavior. The history should indicate when the child smiled, laughed, held up his or her head, sat, stood, walked, cruised unassisted, put his or her first words together, spoke in complete sentences, and rode a tricycle. Inquiries should be made as to when handedness was established.

If the child is in school, where appropriate, information should be obtained from the classroom teacher or from multiple behavioral indices used by the school, such as the Teacher's Questionnaire for Behavioral Assessment or the Connors Scale for

Hyperactivity. All medications the child has received, as well as a listing of all injuries, hospitalizations, and operations, should be recorded.

Suggested Reading

Menkes JH, Sarnat HB, eds. *Child neurology,* 6th edition. Philadelphia: Lippincott Williams & Wilkins, 2000.

Swaiman KF. General aspects of patient neurologic history. In: Swaiman KF, Ashwal S, eds. *Pediatric neurology: principles & practice,* 3rd ed. Vol. 1. St. Louis: Mosby, 1999.

Chapter 4

Neurologic Examination

NEONATAL EXAMINATION

The neonatal examination evaluates the term and preterm infant before 1 month of age. The evaluation of the preterm infant may be particularly vexing. The gestational age of the patient, the lack of developmental norms, and the need for life support systems complicate the performance of an accurate examination. Estimation of gestational age is a more reliable indicator of neurologic maturation than is birth weight.

Assessment of the Preterm Infant

Periods of wakefulness are rare before 28 weeks of gestational age (GA). External stimulation is also necessary to arouse the baby. However, by 32 weeks of GA, external stimulation is usually unnecessary. Periods of wakefulness and somnolence are relatively brief, and they change swiftly. The waking periods of the child at 25 to 30 weeks of gestation are short compared with those of the term infant. The electroencephalogram may be a useful measure of gestational age. Electroencephalographic patterns change quantitatively every 2 weeks from 28 to 40 weeks.

The preterm infant adopts the postures that correspond typically to gestational age. The very young child tends to be hypotonic, and, when the infant is held in a ventral suspension, he or she will not extend the head, arms, or trunk. Although deep tendon reflexes can be obtained in 98% of infants older than 33 weeks of age, these reflexes are difficult to elicit in the preterm child. Changes from hypotonia to the flexor posture of the term infant are manifested first in the legs and then in the arms and head. At 34 weeks of GA, the newborn will assume a frog-like position. By 40 weeks of GA, the frog-like position is lost and the legs should be fully extended. Body tone tends to increase proximally. This is best illustrated by the scarf sign, which is elicited by folding the arm across the chest toward the opposite shoulder. In the preterm infant, the elbow may reach the opposite shoulder, whereas in the term infant the elbow cannot be brought beyond the midline (see Appendix II, Newborn Maturity Rating and Classification).

The postural and righting reflexes cannot be elicited in the 20-week-old preterm infant. Over the next several weeks, the infant will gradually support his or her weight, and, by 34 weeks of GA, a good supporting response, as manifested by postural and righting reflexes, can be obtained. Stretching movements of the limbs may be seen in small preterm infants when they are awake, but this is less common during sleep. The preterm infant may cry to provocation, but crying often occurs when it is unprovoked. By 36 to 37 weeks of GA, the cry is more vigorous, more frequent, and more easily elicited with noxious stimulation.

A pupillary light reflex is not seen before 29 to 30 weeks of GA. At this stage the infant's pupils are usually meiotic, and the palpebral fissure is small. The light reflex becomes more evident by 32 weeks of age. Rudimentary scanning and tracking can be seen in infants who are 31 to 32 weeks of GA. During this time, associated widening of the palpebral fissure is seen. By 36 to 38 weeks of GA, the infant rotates the head to the light and closes his or her eyes forcefully. A doll's eye response is elicited in 28-week-old to 32-week-old preterm infants who have had no neurologic compromise. This reflex is difficult to elicit in the normal infant.

Rooting and sucking reflexes are perfunctory until 34 weeks of GA. In fact, the first act of breathing may be a swallow. The Moro reflex is first present at 24 weeks of GA, but it is not developed until 28 weeks and the infant easily fatigues at this period of time. At 38 weeks of GA, the characteristic response can be elicited. At 28 weeks of GA, the grasp reflex is evident in the fingers but not in the hand. However, by 32 weeks of GA, the palm and fingers may participate in the grasp reflex. The tonic neck reflex cannot be elicited well until approaching term. Some have even suggested this may not be elicited until the first several weeks of life. Automatic walking or the stepping and placing reflexes are not seen until 37 weeks of GA.

As with the general neurologic examination, plotting the rate of head growth is important. The head grows very rapidly in the intrauterine period, as well as during the first year of life. As might be expected, the shape and growth of the head changes markedly in preterm infants. Both the anterior-posterior diameter and the biparietal diameter increase rapidly in preterm infants during the first several months of age. A standard plot of head growth should be used to monitor head growth in the preterm infant. Signs and symptoms of hydrocephalus may not be immediately present, although an increasing rate of head circumference growth, frontal bossing, scaphocephaly, and upward displacement of the external occipital protuberance may suggest hydrocephalus. The maximum velocity of head growth in infants with good caloric intake is found immediately postpartum.

In assessing the preterm child's development, correction for gestation should be taken into account. However, if the development of the preterm infant is normal, it should approximate that of the term infant by the age of 1 year.

Term Infant

The evaluation of the term infant is more informative than is that of the preterm infant. Apgar scores obtained at the time of birth provide an immediate indicator of neurologic distress. The Apgar score, developed in 1953, consists of five different measurements, each of which is given a score of 0 to 2 (see Appendix V). The Apgar is measured at 1, 5, and 10 minutes. Apgar scores above 5 at 5 minutes usually have no long-term consequences, whereas Apgar scores below that number are often associated with significant neurologic abnormalities.

In the immediate newborn period of time, the infant should be assessed for any developmental defects. This includes a search for midline defects of the cranium, face, palate, and spine and for associated neurocutaneous abnormalities. Dermatologic findings of many of the neurocutaneous abnormalities, such as neurofibromatosis and tuberous sclerosis, although they are subtle in infancy, become increasingly obvious during the first decade of life.

Motor Examination

The gross motor abilities of the newborn can be evaluated by observation. The head may potentially be turned to the right for longer periods than to the left. Despite this, term infants when placed in the prone position will invariably clear their airway by turning the head either to the right or left. Failure to clear the airway in the prone position suggests central nervous system abnormalities. Bilateral fisting of the hands with abduction of the thumb into the palm suggests a pyramidal tract disorder. Even in the newborn, the hands should be open 50% of the time. Spontaneous limb movements may be asymmetric with a rapid jerking quality. Unsustained clonus should never be considered problematic. Diminished movement of an arm may indicate a brachial plexus injury, with or without associated Horner syndrome. Similarly, failure to move one arm or leg may indicate a hemiparesis. Abnormalities of respiration may suggest anterior horn cell disease. The absence of neck muscles suggests either anterior horn cell disease or spinal cord injury.

Head Circumference

Measurement of the head circumference is axiomatic in all examinations. A large or small head always suggests neurologic disease. Serial measurement is an index of brain volume *and* brain mass. The impetus to head growth is stress on the parietal dura by the underlying growth of the brain. The shape of the head influences the measurement of the head circumference. The more circular the head, the smaller the head circumference is, whereas a noncircular, dolichocephalic, or scaphocephalic head is associated with a larger head circumference. The head circumference should be plotted on a head growth chart. Concerns should be raised if head growth significantly crosses successive isobars. In this circumstance, possible causes of an enlarged head, such as hydrocephalus, a subdural hematoma, or an intracranial mass, should be raised. The failure of the head to grow along an isobar may suggest microcephaly and either loss of or failure to develop appropriate brain volume.

Infants born to a primiparous mother may have some increase in head size because of scalp and subcutaneous edema. Vacuum extraction often results in a caput succedaneum. This is usually transient, and it goes away within a period of 1 week. On the other hand, infants delivered by cesarean section have relatively round symmetric heads. A caput, unlike a cephalohematoma, extends over two or more cranial bones, and it is not limited by the cranial sutures. The anterior fontanelle is palpable at birth, either concave or flat in relation to the surrounding cranium. The posterior fontanelle may be open or closed. The anterior fontanelle usually closes by 18 months of age, whereas the posterior fontanelle closes by 9 months of age. In patients with craniosynostosis, suture lines cannot be palpated and the fontanelles are closed. The head fails to grow perpendicular to the line of closure. For example, sagittal synostosis associated with premature closure of the sagittal suture is associated with increased growth in an anterior parietal diameter and resultant scaphocephaly. Plagiocephaly occurs in the presence of unilateral coronal synostosis.

Deep Tendon Reflexes and Tone

Motor evaluation of the infant consists of an assessment of tone and strength. Tone is generally defined as resistance to passive movement. In the newborn infant, tone tends to be increased proximally and to be decreased distally. A normal infant held in the horizontal position will raise his or her chest and neck muscles and will extend the legs (Landau reflex). The hypotonic infant, on the other hand, will flex the head; the thorax will be draped over the examiner's hand, and the legs will hang limply from the torso. In the vertical position, flexor tone should be elicited and the legs should not extend, or, if they do extend, the extensor tone should be easily broken when weight is applied over the pelvis. An early sign of pyramidal dysfunction is suggested if an infant's weight cannot be broken over the hips with pressure applied to the pelvis when the infant is held in a vertical position. The hypotonic infant will loosely slide through the examiner's hands. Conversely, infants with increased tone may be opisthotonic with hyperextension of neck and spine.

Tone may be decreased in neuromuscular conditions, such as spinal muscular atrophy, myasthenia gravis, and neonatal myotonic dystrophy, or in congenital myopathies. Crying tends to stimulate movement or motion, and it is associated with increased tone. A noxious stimulus may be associated with crying and an abrupt improvement of tone. These maneuvers point away from a neuromuscular problem and suggest that the difficulty may be central in origin.

Tremulousness may be perfectly benign. Excessive tremulousness may suggest perinatal asphyxia, metabolic developmental abnormalities, or drug withdrawal.

Deep tendon reflexes are usually symmetric; even if they are not elicited, they should not cause concern unless they are asymmetric. Similarly, plantar responses should not be considered abnormal unless they are asymmetric. Ankle clonus is frequently elicited in the newborn; it is generally less than 8 to 12 beats and is rarely of neurologic consequence. Sustained ankle clonus, however, may suggest involvement of the corticospinal tracts.

Cranial Nerves

As in the older child, the cranial nerves should be systematically evaluated. The second cranial nerve can easily be evaluated. That the examiner is a good funduscopist is axiomatic. Evaluation of the optic fundi may require cycloplegics. The retina should be assessed for macular changes and abnormalities of the disk. Retinal hemorrhages are commonly seen after a vaginal delivery, despite the absence of trauma. The color of the optic disk in a newborn is grayish white. The hypoplastic nerve, however, is ivory in color. The infant will turn toward a light of moderate intensity and will fix on the examiner's face, but the eyes will not pursue through 180 degrees. Although newborn visual acuity is difficult to assess, most agree that the newborn has significant visual acuity. Newborns will respond to large colored objects.

The pupils should be symmetric, and they should respond equally to light. The presence of ptosis, meiosis, or abnormalities of the palpebral fissure should be evaluated. Heterochromia should be ascertained. The iris is lightest at birth, and it subsequently becomes increasingly pigmented over the course of the first year of life.

The extraocular muscles should be monitored when the infant is either feeding or lying quietly. With patience and perseverance, the infant may follow an object in a lateral direction. Opticokinetic nystagmus can be elicited using a large striped cloth or a drum. The doll's eye movement should be symmetric. If it is asymmetric, an abnormality of the third or sixth cranial nerve should be suspected.

Facial movements should be observed during crying. Asymmetry of the mouth may indicate an abnormality of the seventh cranial nerve. Depression of the mouth with crying is normal, and its absence suggests an abnormality on the side of the mouth that is not depressed. A congenital absence of one of the facial muscles may be associated with asymmetric sucking or movement of the mouth. This is usually caused by hypoplasia of the depressor muscles of the angle of the mouth. The seventh cranial nerve is responsible for the superficial muscles of facial expression and lip closure.

Hearing can be assessed by brainstem auditory-evoked responses, by placing the patient in a sound booth, or by free field testing. A gross and less reliable technique is to determine whether or not the infant can be stilled by a 512–cycle-per-second tuning fork. While the patient is crying, the tuning fork is presented to either ear. If the infant quiets or turns to the direction of the tuning fork, one can assume that hearing is intact on that side. Sucking and swallowing are complex acts involving the ninth and tenth cranial nerves. Observing the child rotate the neck laterally tests the eleventh nerve. Loss of tongue bulk suggests twelfth nerve difficulties.

EXAMINATION OF THE CHILD OVER 2 YEARS OF AGE

The neurologic examination of the child over 2 years of age is similar to that of an adult, but it must be qualified by a knowledge of developmental milestones. Unlike the adult, failure to acquire expected milestones implies a loss of function. The young child is continuously refining and adapting to new neurologic skills. For instance, vision and hearing become more acute even beyond 2 years of age. The ability to whistle, to use the tongue and palate, and to speak are all developmental milestones. Similarly, hopping, skipping, running, jumping, and climbing all relate to maturation of the gross motor system. Drawing, throwing, cutting with scissors, painting, and writing are developmental indices suggesting the appropriate acquisition of fine motor skills. Thus, the recognition that, in addition to loss of function, failure to acquire appropriate milestones may suggest disease and/or neurologic compromise is important.

As with any clinical assessment, the examination begins with an accurate history followed by observation of the patient. Thus, an understanding of emerging behavioral patterns that present over the first several years of life, as well as a rudimentary knowledge of what is expected of a child during the school years, is important. The child should be engaged in the examination with questions directed to his or her level of intellectual and behavioral ability, and the responses should be compared with known norms.

Although the examination—specifically, that of the cranial nerves—may not be elicited in an organized manner, when it is finally described, it should be organized in a sequential manner for the best presentation of any elicited abnormalities.

Cranial Nerves

Olfactory Nerve

The first cranial nerve (olfactory nerve) is rarely impaired in childhood, and it is only evaluated in a rudimentary manner. Anosmia may occur in children with respiratory infections or in those who have suffered head trauma, and it may involve neoplasms of the frontal lobe or cubiform plate. The child is asked to assess pleasant smells through each nostril while the other is manually occluded.

Visual Pathway

Examination of the optic pathway begins with an assessment of visual acuity. Testing should be performed in appropriately lit rooms. The child is asked to recognize objects of various sizes, shapes, and colors. After 4 to 5 years of age, the E-test is useful (Fig. 4.1). The child is asked to identify the direction that the arms of an "E" are pointing. As with the adult, the visual fields are assessed by confrontation with a small 3-mm white or red object or the examiner's fingers presented to each quadrant of the visual field. Directing the child's gaze first into one field and then into the other can assess visual fields.

The disk of the older child, as in the adult, is often salmon colored, differing from the pale coloration of the infant's disk. Optic atrophy may appear both centrally and peripherally, and it is accompanied by decreased vascularity around the disk margin. In patients with optic atrophy from amblyopia, color vision tends to be preserved. The disk must be identified for accurate exclusion of papilledema. Papilledema is characterized by blurring of the disk margins, hyperemia of the nerve head, an increase in the size of the cecal scotoma, and desaturation for the color red. Disks should also be evaluated for hemorrhages, exudates, and abnormal pigmentation.

Pupillary Response

The diameter, contour, and responsivity of pupils to light should be recorded. In Horner syndrome, the upper lid may cover over

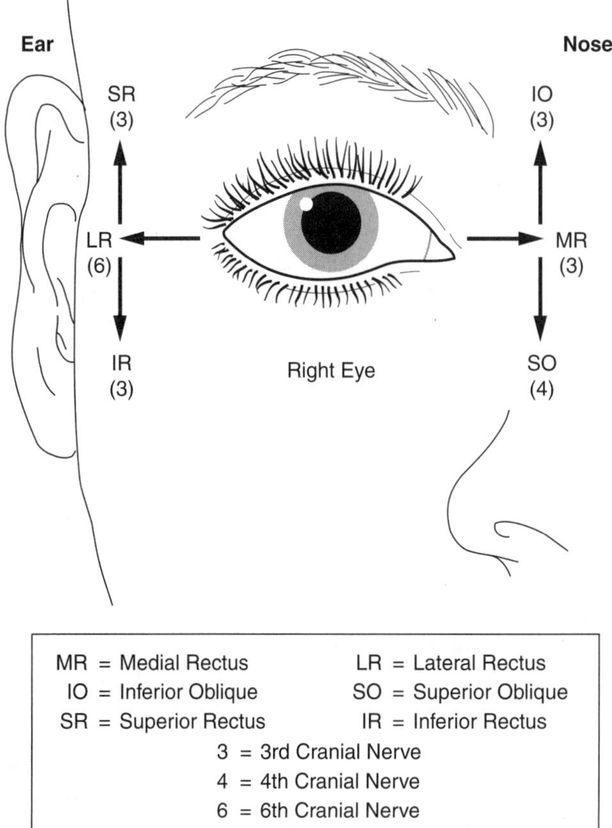

FIGURE 4.1 Primary direction of gaze of extraocular eye muscles.

half the pupil; the syndrome is associated with a miotic pupil and lack of sweating on the ipsilateral side. A fixed dilated pupil usually implies intracranial involvement of the third cranial nerve.

The Marcus-Gunn pupil or an afferent pupillary reflex suggests abnormalities of the papillomacular bundle. This is readily elicited in patients with unilateral optic atrophy in which vision is intact on one side when compared with the other. The reflex is elicited by alternately applying a light source to the normal eye and then swinging the light source to the contralateral abnormal eye. A light applied to the normal eye will cause ipsilateral and contralateral contraction of the pupils. However, when light is applied to the abnormal eye, that eye will appear to dilate paradoxically if the afferent reflex is lost. Although much can be learned at the bedside, when doubt about visual integrity is present, a formal ophthalmologic evaluation is required.

Extraocular Muscles (Fig. 4.1)

The third, fourth, and sixth cranial nerves control the extraocular muscles. Because these muscles act as both rotators and primary directional movers of the eye, the muscle should be put in a plane of gaze where the action of the muscle is in one primary direction only. The third cranial nerve innervates the medial rectus, the superior and inferior rectus, the inferior oblique, and the elevator of the lid. The fourth cranial nerve innervates the superior oblique muscle, and the sixth cranial nerve innervates the lateral rectus. The extraocular muscles are best evaluated when the patient is asked to look medially or laterally and then up and down. On the medial gaze, the primary depressor of the eye is the superior oblique, the adductor of the eye is the medial rectus, and the elevator of the eye is the inferior oblique. On lateral gaze, the depressor of the eye is the inferior rectus, the abductor of the eye is the lateral rectus, and the elevator of the eye is the superior rectus.

Heterophoria refers to the breaking of fusion when the eyes are on near or far objects during fixation. Alternately covering and uncovering each eye forces fixation of the uncovered eye and uncovers the presence of a heterophoria. Exophoria is the predisposition of the eye to diverge laterally, whereas esophoria implies medial deviation. If noncongruence is seen during binocular vision without a cover and uncover test, this is termed heterotropia. Although phorias commonly occur and may be brought out with sickness or may be seen in the myopic individual, tropias often suggest abnormalities of extraocular muscle function.

In testing for diplopia, the clinician must remember that objects have a tendency to be further apart when the test object is moved away from the midline of the body, either vertically or horizontally. With use of the Red Glass Test, the patient should report a separation of objects when he or she is looking in the direction of action of the affected muscle. The false image is the one that is the most peripheral, and it represents the object that is seen by the abnormal eye. Volitional turning of the head accompanies paresis of the lateral rectal muscles. Tilting of the head toward the shoulder of the opposite side is seen in patients with a superior oblique palsy.

Opticokinetic Nystagmus Response

Opticokinetic nystagmus response is useful in evaluating the eye movements of inattentive young children. A tape with stripes or figures is drawn before the child in both horizontal and vertical directions from one field to the contralateral field. If a tracking nystagmus is elicited, the child will track the object in the direction of the tape. When the stripe goes out of the field of vision, the child rapidly refixates in the reverse direction. Absence of such movements may occur in the presence of visual loss, abnormal saccadic eye movements, or inattention. This is a useful test for excluding functional difficulties from clinical blindness. Children with congenital nystagmus may or may not have an absent opticokinetic response.

Nystagmus

Nystagmus may be jerk, vertical, or rotatory. Pendular nystagmus suggests rhythmic abnormalities that are equal in all planes of gaze, and it is associated with either cerebellar or retinal disease, whereas jerk nystagmus consists of a slow and fast phase and it refers to abnormalities of the vestibular system. The most common cause of nystagmus in children is induced by centrally acting medications, such as anticonvulsants. Vertical nystagmus, unlike horizontal nystagmus, is primarily seen with abnormalities of the brainstem. Nystagmus may suggest either end-organ or intrinsic disease of the nervous system. Vertical nystagmus, bilateral nystagmus on lateral gaze, primary position nystagmus on horizontal gaze, and nonfatigable positional nystagmus all suggest intrinsic abnormalities of the brainstem. Primary position nystagmus is associated with abnormalities of the pontomesocephalic junction; downbeating small amplitude primary position nystagmus and ocular myoclonus suggest a medullary lesion. Abnormalities of the median longitudinal fasciculus are associated with conversion retraction nystagmus and internuclear ophthalmoplegia. Seesaw nystagmus localizes the pathology to the diencephalon.

Fifth Cranial Nerve

The fifth cranial nerve is divided into the following three segments: the ophthalmic, maxillary, and mandibular divisions. All three have sensory function, whereas the mandibular portion of the fifth cranial nerve is both motor and sensory. Feeling the temporalis muscle bulk can assess motor function. Abnormalities consist of atrophy and scalloping of the temporal fossa. The mass or muscle bulk is assessed by palpation over the muscle belly with the mouth firmly closed, whereas muscle strength is elicited by having the patient open and move the mouth from side to side. The jaw reflex, both afferent and efferent, tests the integrity of the fifth cranial nerve. The reflex may be overactive in the presence of supranuclear lesions and absent in the presence of peripheral lesions.

Seventh Cranial Nerve (See Fig. 8.4)

The seventh cranial nerve, like the fifth, is both sensory and motor. The nerve provides sensation to the anterior two-thirds of the tongue and innervates the lacrimal and salivary glands, initiating taste. The main function of the nerve is motor to the muscles of superficial expression. The facial nerve divides into the following five branches as it exits the cranial fossa through the stylomastoid foramen: temporal, zygomatic, buccal, mandibular, and cervical. This results in the ability to wrinkle the forehead, to close the eye forcefully, and to elevate the corner of the mouth. In a hemispheric lesion, facial nerve impairment produces paresis of the muscles involving the lower face with drooping of the corner of the mouth, disappearance of the nasal labial fold, and variable widening of the palpebral fissure. In a peripheral injury, the branches of the nerve can be affected singularly or it may involve the entire nerve. In branch lesions, movement of the muscles of the forehead, face, and nose and closure of the eye may not be uniformly involved. Although taste in part is subserved by the chorda tympani nerve, which comes from the fifth cranial nerve, its path traverses the anatomic pathway of the facial nerve for a short distance beyond the geniculate ganglion, and hence it may be involved in lesions distal to the geniculate ganglia.

Eighth Cranial Nerve

The eighth cranial nerve tests auditory and vestibular function. Gross hearing loss can be assessed at the bedside, but more refined testing is obtained in a sound booth or by brainstem auditory-evoked responses. A whispered sound should be presented to the involved ear while the contralateral ear is masked with either rubbing of the fingers or other forms of white noise. The ability to hear a whispered sound presented to the ear usually implies hearing at a minimum of 30 decibels. All children who are delayed in speech should be tested for hearing loss. Although older children can cooperate with formal audiometric testing, younger children can be assessed in an auditory booth using free field testing. An auditory sound is presented from multiple directions. The child is expected to turn in the direction of the heard sound. Brainstem auditory-evoked response is used as a nonvolitional determinant of hearing.

Clinical history and caloric testing is used to assess vestibular function. Complaints of nausea, attacks of vertigo, or unexplained vomiting suggest abnormalities of vestibular function. Caloric testing is determined by using a cold water stimulus of 30°C and a warm water stimulus of 44°C. The patient is placed in the supine position with the head flexed to 30 degrees. Either warm or cold water is injected for a period of 30 seconds into one external canal at a time. The fast component with cold water stimulation is directed toward the opposite ear, whereas the fast component with warm water stimulation is directed toward the ipsilateral ear.

Bulbar Cranial Nerves (IX Through XII)

The ninth and tenth cranial nerves innervate the larynx, pharynx, and palate. Unilateral paresis of the palate causes an ipsilateral droop or drape sign. Bilateral involvement causes a flat, soft palate. The gag reflex is obtained by stimulating the posterior pharyngeal mucosa. Both the ninth and tenth cranial nerves are responsible for a gag reflex. The larynx can be studied more appropriately under direct laryngoscopy or by fluoroscopy. Evaluation of hoarseness and dystonia requires a more detailed examination.

The eleventh cranial nerve innervates the trapezius and sternocleidomastoid muscles. The trapezius muscle is assessed when the child is asked to shrug his or her shoulders against resistance. Atrophy of the muscle may be readily evaluated. Asking the patient to turn his or her head to the contralateral side of the muscle involved assesses the sternocleidomastoid muscle. The head is turned to the side while pressure is applied to the contralateral chin. The muscle bulk on the contralateral side from that of the chin pressure is readily palpable and evaluated.

The hypoglossal nerve (cranial nerve XII) tests the integrity of the tongue. Atrophy and fasciculation are readily seen with involvement of the hypoglossal nerve or nucleus. This is best evaluated with the mouth open and the tongue nonprotruded. A protruded tongue will deviate toward the involved side, whereas a tongue in the mouth will deviate toward the contralateral side. Involvement of the tongue causes dysarthria. Twelfth nerve abnormalities can result from either supranuclear bulbar palsy, nuclear involvement, or involvement of the nerve itself.

Sensation

The evaluation of sensation in the child may be a tour de force. Vibration and touch are readily elicited. Touch can be assessed by either single or double-simultaneous stimulation. Evaluation of pain, on the other hand, is difficult, and it may present a diagnostic challenge. The child should be reassured that a pinprick will not be painful, and the approach should be gentle and nonthreatening. Segmental dermatomes and segmental sensory loss are similar to the adult (see Chapter 2).

Motor

Motor examination tests reveal tone, bulk, and strength. Tone is defined as resistance to movement, and it may be normal, increased, or decreased. Dystonia is defined as an abnormal attitude of posture.

Strength is graded on a scale of one to five as follows: 5, normal power; 4, ability to generate power with moderate resistance; 3, ability to elicit power against gravity; 2, ability to elicit resistance with gravity eliminated; 1, contraction of the muscle; 0, no strength at all. Testing the function of specific muscles or muscle groups is beyond the scope of this manual. The reader is referred to either standard textbooks of neurology or to the *Medical Research Counsel memorandum on aid to the investigation of peripheral nerve injuries,* which is published in London. This small manual beautifully demonstrates testing of isolated muscle groups.

Movement

Gait and station involve both motor and cerebellar function. The child is asked to walk forward and backward, both on his or her toes and heels, and to tandem walk. The child is also asked to stand with his or her feet together with the eyes both open and closed and to get up from a lying or sitting position to an upright posture. Observation should be made as to whether the gait is wide or narrow based and if reciprocal movements of the arms and legs are seen. Posture in the arms and legs should be noted when he or she is walking, as well as whether the abnormalities of gait involving an affected limb are either proximal or distal. Asymmetries are intensified when the child is asked to run or to toe walk. The abnormalities can be characterized as spastic, athetotic, dystonic, hypotonic, or cerebellar.

Cerebellum

Axial or Trunk Assessment

The cerebellum primarily maintains the normal synergy and fluidity of muscle activity. Cerebellar deficits are notable in abnormalities of equilibrium, posture, and voluntary movement. In testing the cerebellum, a disruption in the normal synergy of movement, whether axial or appendicular, is determined. Axial abnormalities are noted primarily when the child is sitting or walking. The child should be asked to stand in front of the examiner, to walk both forward and backward, to walk on his or her toes, and to tandem walk along a straight line. Hopping, skipping, and jumping may also bring out unilateral abnormalities. In the normal child, gait is characterized by less than 3 to 4 mm of one foot clearing the other. However, in cerebellar disease, the gait may be wide based, and the inability to pivot around a narrow base is lost. If gait is wide based, the child cannot turn on a narrow base, or the gait is broken up into its component parts, abnormality of the vermis of the cerebellum is suggested.

Appendicular or Limb Appraisal

In testing appendicular abnormalities, attempts are made to evaluate the fine motor skills. The patient is asked to perform finger–nose and heel–shin movements. Abnormalities are noted primarily in proximal, rather than distal, musculature. The greatest abnormality in fluidity of movement is when the arm is abducted and the finger is brought to the nose. Similarly, the greatest defect is seen when the leg is abducted and the heel is placed on the knee before running it down the pretibial surface.

Errors in estimation of amplitude of movement are termed dysmetria, whereas abnormalities in alternating movements are termed dysdiadochokinesis. In assessing these, the clinician should also elicit abnormalities in rhythmic finger and foot tapping. Change in muscle tone may also suggest cerebellar function, because the cerebellum primarily helps to maintain the functional resting tone of the muscle. Hypotonia may suggest abnormalities of this system. Similarly, because normal cerebellar function primarily inhibits the cerebral motor systems, an abnormal rebound phenomenon may suggest cerebellar problems. Rebound is elicited by asking the patient with the arm flexed to develop resistance to an examiner's attempt to extend the arm. When resistance is rapidly diminished, the flexed arm may fly with considerable force into the examiner's face or chest. The rebound phenomenon has been recognized as an example of a cerebellar abnormality for close to a century.

General Features of Cerebellar Dysfunction

Cerebellar gait is characterized as staggering, wide-based, unsteady, lurching movements with a breakdown of the normal synergy of walking. The Romberg test indicates dorsal column function; it is not primarily a test of cerebellar function. Scanning or staccato speech may also reflect cerebellar abnormalities. Nystagmus, although this is considered a cerebellar function, is usually not seen with primary disease of the cerebellum, but it can be seen with spinal cerebellar degenerations or the involvement of tracts that go in and out of the cerebellum. When nystagmus is present in cerebellar hemisphere lesions, it tends to be coarser and slower when directed toward the side of the lesion and finer and less intense when directed toward the opposite side.

OVERALL ASSESSMENT

Once the neurologic examination is obtained, the collected information should be assessed in an organized fashion. An attempt should be made to determine whether a single anatomic location of the abnormality can be determined. This can be assessed by evaluating both the horizontal and vertical location of the lesion, which helps to determine where in the nervous system groups of anatomical abnormalities exist in proximity. Motor, sensory, and cerebellar systems project up and down the neuraxis cord extending from the cortex to the spinal cord. Cranial nerves, peripheral nerves, and vegetative functions, on the other hand, tend to be confined to more localized areas within the central nervous system.

Suggested Reading

Fenichel GM. The neurologic examination of the newborn. *Brain Dev* 1993;15:403–410.

Fenichel GM. *Clinical pediatric neurology: a signs and symptoms approach,* 4th ed. Philadelphia: WB Saunders, 2001.

Paine RS. Neurologic examination of infants and children. *Pediatr Clin North Am* 1960;7:41.

Paine RS. The evolution of infantile postural reflexes in the presence of chronic brain syndromes. *Dev Med Child Neurol* 1964;6:345.

Paine RS, Oppe TW. *Neurological examination of children.* London: William Heinemann, 1966.

Swaiman KF, Ashwal S. *Pediatric neurology: principles and practice.* St. Louis: Mosby, 1999.

Chapter 5

Floppy Infant

Case

A 6-month-old infant presents with the history of being unable to sit. She was normal until 3 months of age, when she seemed to be getting weaker. By 6 months, she could no longer turn over or reach for objects. On examination, she was alert and playful. She was extremely hypotonic with poor head control and a tendency to lie in a "frog-leg" position. Sensation was normal. She was weak, and she could not generate tone. Her deep tendon reflexes were absent, and the tongue fasciculated.

Diagnosis

Infantile spinal muscular atrophy (SMA)

"Floppy infant" refers to an infant less than 1 year of age who is hypotonic and whose examination is characterized by the following signs:

- Displays poor head control when pulled to a sitting position;
- Forms the posture of a "C" when held in ventral suspension;
- Lies in a frog-leg position (abduction of legs, with the lateral surface of the thighs on the table).

A infant may be hypotonic due to **a lesion in either the central or peripheral nervous system** as follows:

- Brain
- Spinal cord

- Peripheral nerve
- Neuromuscular junction
- Muscle
- Generalized (e.g., Down syndrome, hypothyroidism)

The **history** is important in identifying the level of the lesion.

- Is the condition static or progressive? Is delay in attaining milestones or the loss of previously attained skills observed?
- If the condition is progressive, what is the tempo?
- Does infant have adaptive, as well as motor, abnormalities? (This suggests cortical involvement rather than peripheral nervous system disease.)
- Does infant have a history of seizures? (This suggests cortical involvement.)
- Are other medical problems present? (Their presence suggests a generalized metabolic disorder.)
- Does the infant show poor feeding? (The condition may be bulbar or pseudobulbar.)
- Is infant extremely irritable? (This is typical in Krabbe disease.)

HISTORY

Problems with Obtaining History

- Young age, so milestones are limited.
- Selective memory, often wishful thinking.

Birth History

- Movements *in utero:* the infant who does not move normally *in utero* may have a neuromuscular problem.
- Polyhydramnios: this suggests that the infant had abnormal swallowing *in utero.*
- Delivery: a difficult delivery may suggest a central cause for the infant's hypotonia, but a difficult delivery does not exclude the presence of degenerative disease.

FAMILY HISTORY

Items of Interest

- Miscarriages
- Neurologic diseases

Problems with Family History

Some patients with neurologic disease may be unaware that they have a neurologic disease. For example, a mother with myotonic dystrophy may be unaware of her diagnosis until her infant is born with neonatal myotonic dystrophy.

PHYSICAL EXAMINATION

General

The following should be assessed:

- Cornea (may be abnormal in mucopolysaccharidoses).
- High-pitched cry (may suggest cerebral dysfunction).
- Respiratory pattern (abdominal breathing suggests neuromuscular disease).
- Joints (arthrogryposis multiplex may be associated with infantile SMA or another form of intrauterine neuromuscular disease).
- Skin (dry skin may suggest hypothyroidism).
- Hair (blond kinky hair may suggest Menkes syndrome).
- Heart (cardiomegaly may suggest Pompe disease).
- Abdomen (hepatosplenomegaly can be associated with Niemann-Pick or other storage diseases).

Neurologic Examination

- *Head circumference.* An infant with a normal head circumference at birth and who, at 6 months, is below the 5th percentile may have had perinatal asphyxia. The infant with a head circumference that is crossing percentiles may have storage disease.
- *Socialization.* The child who is interactive and age appropriate from a socialization point of view likely has a problem outside of the brain. This can be an important inclusionary or exclusionary finding.
- *Cranial nerve II.* Cherry-red spot may suggest a storage disease, such as Tay-Sachs disease or metachromatic leukodystrophy; optic atrophy may suggest Krabbe disease or metachromatic leukodystrophy.
- *Cranial nerves II and III.* Abnormal eye movements and a lack of pupillary light reflex may suggest infantile botulism.
- *Cranial nerve VII.* Facial diparesis may suggest neonatal myotonic dystrophy.

- *Cranial nerves IX and X.* Difficulties with swallowing and handling secretions may suggest either neuromuscular problems or suprabulbar palsy.
- *Cranial nerve XII.* Fasciculation of the tongue suggests infantile SMA.

Motor

- *Decreased tone but normal strength.* Just because an infant is hypotonic, this does not mean the infant is weak. The infant who is floppy with normal strength suggests a cerebral cause, such as a static encephalopathy (cerebral palsy).
- *Decreased tone and weak.* The infant who is floppy *and* weak has abnormalities of the final common pathway (from the anterior horn cell to the nerve, neuromuscular junction, and muscle).
- *The floppy infant who can generate tone.* This suggests that the final common pathway is intact; more likely, the etiology is central.
- *Distribution of weakness.* Proximal muscle weakness is more suggestive of either infantile SMA or myopathy, whereas distal weakness is more typically seen in neuropathies. Myotonic dystrophy is worse distally than proximally.
- *Fisting.* The child who has "cortical thumbs" suggests a primary intracranial process.

Deep Tendon Reflexes

- Increased, clonus, Babinski (brain, spinal cord)
- Normal (muscle, neuromuscular junction)—Absent in botulism
- Absent (anterior horn cell, roots, nerve)

LOCATION OF THE LESION

Is It in the Brain?

The most common cause of floppy infant syndrome is static encephalopathy (atonic type). The course is static and nonprogressive. The delivery may have been complicated by anoxia and fetal distress. Many children have mental retardation, often with microcephaly and seizures. The infant is floppy but not weak, and he or she can generate tone. Reflexes are increased with Babinski responses. Sensation is normal.

Other cerebral causes of floppy infant are chromosomal abnormalities, such as Prader-Willi syndrome. The condition is static and nonprogressive. The syndrome includes mental retardation, hypogonadism, obesity, and an abnormality of chromosome 15.

Infants with a degenerative disease, such as Tay-Sachs disease, may initially present as floppy infants, but the course is one of progressive deterioration. Mental regression and seizures are common. Infants are usually floppy but not weak. Reflexes are present, and sensation is normal. Funduscopic examination will reveal a cherry red spot. Diagnosis is made by assessment of hexosaminidase A.

Other degenerative brain diseases, such as Krabbe and metachromatic leukodystrophy, affect the brain *and* peripheral nerves. Regression of motor and adaptive milestones is seen. Infants may be floppy and weak, with a loss of deep tendon reflexes but upgoing toes. Funduscopic examination may reveal optic atrophy. The evaluation includes lysosomal enzymes and magnetic resonance imaging of the brain.

Is It in the Spinal Cord?

Spinal cord transection typically occurs with breech presentation. Depending on the level of the transection, the infant will initially be hypotonic and weak below the level of the transection. Over time, spasticity typically develops. Reflexes may also be absent initially due to spinal shock, but they will eventually be increased with evidence of clonus and Babinski reflex. Urinary retention will be present. A sensory level is present. Typically, intelligence is preserved. Evaluation includes magnetic resonance imaging and x-rays of the spine.

Is It in the Anterior Horn Cell?

Poliomyelitis is a viral illness that affects the anterior horn cells in an asymmetric fashion. Typically, a prodrome of a febrile illness is observed. The bulbar and respiratory muscles may be affected. The deep tendon reflexes are absent, and sensation is normal. Diagnosis is made by cerebrospinal fluid analysis and viral cultures.

Infantile SMA, type I, is an autosomal recessive illness characterized by a progressive deterioration in motor function. The infant's cognition is normal. The tongue fasciculates, but no evidence of facial diparesis is seen. The infant is hypotonic and weak without reflexes. Sensation is normal. Abdominal breathing is characteristic. Diagnosis is made by DNA analysis (chromosome 5q).

Acute Infantile Spinal Muscular Atrophy, Type I

Onset

- Birth to 6 months
- May begin intrauterine (decreased fetal movements)

Symptoms

- Good social interaction
- Weakness: proximal is greater than distal
- Hypotonia
- Sensation: normal
- Facial movement: normal
- Extraocular movement: normal
- Fasciculations of the tongue
- Paradoxical respirations (weakness of the intercostal muscles)
- Relentless progression
- Death from aspiration and/or pneumonia
- Mortality of 90%

Evaluation

- Creatine phosphokinase: normal to mildly increased
- Electromyogram (EMG)
  - Fibrillations and fasciculations at rest
  - Increased mean amplitude of motor unit potentials
  - Motor nerve conductor velocity: normal
- Muscle biopsy—grouped fiber atrophy
- DNA analysis (can be performed *in utero*)

Pathophysiology

- The anterior horn cells and motor nuclei of the brainstem are progressively lost.

Genetics

- Autosomal recessive
- Defect in chromosome 5q

Treatment

- Pulmonary toilet
- Gastrostomy
- Prevent contractures with vigorous physical therapy—range of motion exercises

Chronic Infantile Spinal Muscular Atrophy, Type II

Genetics

- Autosomal recessive
- Defect in chromosome 5q

Onset

- Six to 18 months (may begin at 3 months)

Symptoms

- Normal up to 6 to 8 months of age
- Symmetric proximal weakness: legs more than the arms
- Deep tendon reflexes: decreased or absent
- Most sit, stand; some walk
- Face not affected
- Extraocular muscles spared
- Progression slow in infancy, then stabilizes for years
- Survival to adult life
- Contractures, equinovarus posture common
- Minipolymyoclonus of fingers

Evaluation

- Creatine phosphokinase normal
- EMG: same as SMA, type I
- Muscle biopsy
  - Grouped fiber atrophy
  - No type I fiber hypertrophy
- DNA analysis

Juvenile Spinal Muscular Atrophy, Type III

Genetics

- Defect in chromosome 5q
- Autosomal recessive with only rare dominant forms

Onset

- Older than 18 months of age
- May present in late childhood or adolescence

Symptoms

- Lumbar lordosis, genu recurvatum
- Gait instability with second-degree proximal weakness: waddle
- Calf hypertrophy: may or may not be present
- Slowly progressive
- No extraocular muscle involvement
- Deep tendon reflexes: absent or diminished
- May have tremor in hands
- Scoliosis
- May continue to walk
- May have normal life expectancy

Evaluation

- Creatine phosphokinase: two to four times normal
- EMG
  - Fasciculations, fibrillations, sharp waves in 50% of patients
  - Motor nerve conduction delayed late in course
- Muscle biopsy—grouped fiber atrophy with groups of atrophic fibers that are adjacent to fibers that are normal or hypertrophied (type I)
- DNA analysis

Differential Diagnosis of Spinal Muscular Atrophy, Type III

- Limb girdle dystrophy
- Amyotrophic lateral sclerosis (SMA III has no long tract signs)

Is It in the Peripheral Nerve?

Guillain-Barré syndrome can occur in infancy; it presents as a subacute deterioration in motor function. The infant is hypotonic and weak, and the intellect is preserved. The cranial nerves may be affected, especially the facial nerve. Reflexes are absent. No sensory level may be present, but loss of proprioception and vibration may occur. Diagnosis is made by cerebrospinal fluid analysis, which reveals a cytoalbumino disassociation.

Is It at the Neuromuscular Junction?

Botulism may cause an infant to develop subacute weakness. Often, an infant has eaten tainted honey. The child is typically constipated. Infants with this syndrome are hypotonic and weak with absent reflexes and normal sensation. Extraocular movements are affected, and the pupils are large and poorly reactive. Ptosis is often present. Bulbar weakness may make feeding difficult. Diagnosis is made by the identification of botulinum spores in the stool.

Neonatal myasthenia gravis occurs in 10% of infants born to myasthenic mothers. The infants are hypotonic and weak with respiratory compromise, facial involvement, and difficulty with feeding is common. Reflexes are present, and sensation is preserved. Diagnosis is usually clear due to the presence of the disease in the mother, but, in doubtful cases, a trial of neostigmine is indicated. Improvement is seen in the first 3 to 4 weeks of life as maternal antibodies are cleared from the infant's blood.

Toxic Neuromuscular Disorders

Hypermagnesemia may cause hypotonia in the newborn whose mother has been treated with magnesium for preeclampsia. Other toxic causes include aminoglycosides, which may cause neuromuscular blockade.

Is It in the Muscle? (See Chapter 9)

Neonatal myotonic dystrophy occurs in infants born to mothers with myotonic dystrophy. Often the mothers are unaware of their own diagnosis. The infants are hypotonic and weak with a characteristic facial diparesis (inverted "V" mouth). Sensation is normal, and the reflexes are intact. These infants may have respiratory compromise, and their feet have a pes cavus deformity. Diagnosis is made by performing an EMG on the mother.

Congenital myopathies vary in their severity, course, and prognosis. Infants typically present as floppy infants who are weak, but they have preserved reflexes and normal sensation. Most have normal facies as in central core disease, but others may have a facial diparesis (e.g., centronuclear myopathy and nemaline rod myopathy). The diagnosis is made by muscle biopsy.

Pompe disease (acid maltase deficiency) is an example of a metabolic myopathy. It is an autosomal recessive illness with a defective gene on 17q. Infants become floppy either in the postnatal period or by 2 months of age. In addition to severe hypotonia, the child develops congestive heart failure. Glycogen accumulates in brain, spinal cord, and skeletal muscles, which accounts for the hypotonia, depressed deep tendon reflexes, and decreased awareness. Evaluation includes an electrocardiogram (short PR intervals

TABLE 5.1 Differential Diagnosis of Floppy Infant by Location

Diagnosis	Hypotonic	Weak	Adaptive Milestones	DTRs	BABS	Sensory	Progressive	Other
Cerebral								
Static encephalopathy	+	–	Abnormal	↑	+	Normal	–	± Seizure; small head
Leukodystrophy (Krabbe, metachromatic leukodystrophy)	+	±	Abnormal (decline)	–	+	Normal	+	± Seizure; optic atrophy
Spinal cord								
ISMA	+	+	Normal	–	–	Normal	+	Autosomal recessive; tongue fasciculations
Transection	+ (later spastic)	+	Normal	– (shock), then ↑	+	Abnormal (level)	–	Often positive birth history; urinary retention; fecal incontinence
Poliomyelitis	+	+	Normal	–	–	Normal	–	Asymmetric
Peripheral nerves								
Guillain-Barré	+	+	Normal	–	–	No level; ± post column	Subacute onset improves	Postinfectious, often facial diparesis

(*Continued*)

TABLE 5.1 Differential Diagnosis of Floppy Infant by Location (*Continued*)

Diagnosis	Hypotonic	Weak	Adaptive Milestones	DTRs	BABS	Sensory	Progressive	Other
Neuromuscular junction								
Botulism	+	+	Normal	–	–	Normal	Subacute, improves	Constipation; bulbar ↓ EOM, ptosis, ↓ pupillary response
Neonatal myasthenia gravis	+	+	Newborn	+	–	Normal	Improves	Mother—myasthenia gravis + bulbar + respiratory failure; facial weakness, ptosis
Muscle								
Neonatal myotonic dystrophy	+	+	Mental retardation	+	–	Normal	Improves	Facial diparesis; ↓ respiratory, equinovarus; mother myotonic dystrophy in 80%
Congenital myopathy	+	+	Normal	+	–	Normal	Improves	Proximal > distal: facial nemaline rod, centronuclear myopathy

Abbreviations: BABS, Babinski sign; DTR, deep tendon reflexes; EOM, extraocular movement; ISMA, infantile spinal muscular atrophy.

and high QRS complexes) and a fibroblast culture (decreased acid maltase activity). Most die of cardiac failure before 1 year of age.

Multiple systemic causes of hypotonia also are seen, including Down syndrome, hypothyroidism, and congenital laxity of the ligaments. In addition, when infants are ill or septic, they tend to become acutely hypotonic, although this is a transient phenomenon.

EVALUATION

The evaluation of the floppy infant begins first and foremost with a detailed history and physical examination. At the conclusion of this analysis, the level of the lesion should be determined and the appropriate workup should ensue. Neurodiagnostic and metabolic testing should be specific to the disease identified in the differential diagnosis (Table 5.1).

Suggested Reading

Arnon SS, Midura TF, Damus K, et al. Honey and other environmental risk factors for infant botulism. *J Pediatr* 1979;94:331–336.

Bodensteiner JB. Congenital myopathies. *Muscle Nerve* 1994;17:131–144.

Brooke M. *A clinician's view of neuromuscular diseases,* 2nd ed. Baltimore: Williams and Wilkins, 1986.

Brzustowicz LM, Lehner T, Castilla LA, et al. Genetic mapping of childhood-onset spinal muscular atrophy to chromosome 5q11.2-13.3. *Nature* 1990;344:540–541.

Donaldson JO, Penn AS, Lisak RP, et al. Antiacetylcholine receptor antibody in neonatal myasthenia gravis. *Am J Dis Child* 1981;135:222–226.

Dubowitz V. *The floppy infant.* Philadelphia: J.B. Lippincott, 1980.

Dyken PR, Harper PJ. Congenital dystrophia myotonica. *Neurology* 1973; 24:465–473.

Glatman-Freedman A. Infant botulism. *Pediatr Rev* 1996;17:185–186.

Hagenah R, Müller-Jensen A. Botulism: clinical and neurophysiological findings. *Arch Neurol* 1978;217:159–171.

Lefvert AK, Osterman PO. Newborn infants to myasthenic mothers: a clinical study and an investigation of acetylcholine-receptor antibodies in 17 children. *Neurology* 1983;33:133–138.

Martinez BA, Lake BD. Childhood nemaline myopathy: a review of clinical presentation in relation to prognosis. *Dev Med Child Neurol* 1987; 29:815–820.

Norton P, Ellison P, Sulaiman AR, et al. Nemaline myopathy in the neonate. *Neurology* 1983;33:351–356.

Chapter 6

Back Pain

Case

A 4 year old comes into the emergency room with a 24-hour history of irritability and crying. She refuses to walk, complains of stomach pain, and has questionable tenderness over the back. The neurologic examination is unremarkable. The sedimentation rate is elevated. Imaging reveals a collapsed vertebral space with some epidural compression.

Diagnosis

Discitis
The patient was placed on long-term antibiotics and recovered after 6 weeks.

Back pain may result from a variety of causes. In addition to determining the time and tempo of the process, assessing whether the problem involves the spine, roots, nerves, or muscles is important. Axiomatic to the approach is that all back pain of an acute nature is compressive (e.g., blood, pus, tumor) until proven otherwise. Recovery relates directly to the degree and duration of compression.

HISTORY

Time and tempo

- Chronic or acute
- Constant or fluctuating
- Progressive or stable

Focal versus radiating

- Focal pain suggests bone or muscle.
- Radiating pain suggests involvement of roots or nerves.

Aggravated by sitting, standing, or lying

- Pain increased by sitting suggests root pain.
- Pain increased by lying or standing suggests bone pain.

Evaluate whether the pain is sharp, dull, or lancinating.

- Lancinating suggests root entry zone.
- Sharp pain suggests root pain.
- Dull pain suggests bone pain.

EXAMINATION

Deep tendon reflexes—the loss of reflexes localizes the lesion.

- Biceps: C5-6
- Triceps: C6-7
- Patella: L2-4
- Achilles: S1-2
- Test for specific muscle weakness
  - Iliopsoas: L-2 or L-3
  - Quadriceps: L-2, L-3, or L-4
  - Tibialis anterior: L-4 or L-5
  - Gluteus medius: L-5, S-1
  - Extensor hallicus: L-5

COMMON ROOT SYNDROMES

C-5 or C-6 — Pain and sensory loss: shoulder involving the upper arms and the radial side of forearm. Decreased biceps and brachioradialis reflex present. Motor: weak biceps, deltoid, and brachioradialis muscles.

C-7 — Pain and sensory loss in the posterior aspect of the forearm and second and third digits. Absent triceps reflex. Motor: weak triceps and wrist extensors.

C-8 — Pain and sensory loss along the ulnar aspect of the forearm, the lateral aspect of the hand, and the fourth and fifth digits. Motor: weak intrinsic hand muscles.

L-4 — Pain and sensory loss in the anterolateral thigh and knee and the anteromedial leg. Decreased patella reflex. Motor: weak quadriceps and anterior tibialis muscle.

L-5 Pain and sensory loss in the lateral aspect of the lower leg. Motor: weak toe extensors, peroneus longus, and the anterior tibialis (less likely).

S-1 Pain and sensory loss in the buttocks, the posterior thigh, the posterior lateral leg, and lateral foot. Absent to decreased ankle reflex. Motor: weak hamstrings, gluteus maximus, and toe flexors.

CONUS MEDULLARIS VERSUS CAUDA EQUINA LESIONS

Symptoms	*Conus*	*Cauda Equina*
Motor weakness	Symmetric	Asymmetric
Sensory loss	Loss in saddle distribution	Asymmetric or unilateral
Bowel and bladder loss	Early and significant	Late and mild

ACUTE BACK PAIN

Differential Diagnosis

Compressive Disease

Immediate neurosurgical consultation is required. The recovery depends on the degree and the length of time of the compression. In compressive disease, the heavily myelinated tracks (i.e., dorsal columns and corticospinal tracks) are the most vulnerable. Preservation of vibration and position sense suggests possible recovery, whereas loss of these modalities is a poor prognostic sign.

- Hematoma
- Abscess
- Tumor
- Trauma
- Herniated disk

Noncompressive Disease

- Myelitis
- Discitis
- Developmental
  - Spondylitis

  - Spondylolisthesis
  - Spina bifida occulta

Infectious

- Epidural abscess
- Discitis
  - Acute pain
  - Refusal to walk, but no weakness
  - Normal neurologic examination
  - Collapsed vertebrae
  - Epidural mass
- Treatment
  - Surgical drainage, if appropriate
  - Immobilization
  - Prolonged antibiotics for up to 6 weeks—the usual etiology is *Staphylococcus aureus*

CHRONIC BACK PAIN

Differential Diagnosis

Developmental

- Syringomyelia
  - Loss of reflexes
  - Dissociated sensory loss (i.e., intact proprioception and vibration, loss of pain and temperature)
- Hydromyelia
- Kyphoscoliosis
- Tethered cord: check for foot asymmetry, urinary incontinence
- Diplomyelia
- Diastematomyelia
- Lipoma
  - May have tuft of hair
  - Sacral dimple: midline is usually benign; eccentric may be associated with underlying lipoma

Infectious

- Epidural abscess
- Discitis
  - Acute pain

- ◆ Refusal to walk but no weakness
- ◆ Normal neurologic examination
- ◆ Collapsed vertebrae
- ◆ Epidural mass
- ■ Treatment
  - ◆ Surgical drainage, if appropriate
  - ◆ Immobilization
  - ◆ Prolonged antibiotics for up to 6 weeks—the usual etiology is *S. aureus*

Suggested Reading

Batzdorf U. *Syringomyelia: concepts in diagnosis and treatment.* Baltimore: Williams & Wilkins, 1990.

Dawson DM. Entrapment neuropathies of the upper extremities. *N Engl J Med* 1993;329:2013–2018.

Iqbal JB, Bradley N, Macfaul R, et al. Syringomyelia in children: six case reports and review of the literature. *Br J Neurosurg* 1992;6:13–20.

Jansen BR, Hart W, Schreuder O. Discitis in childhood: 12-35-year follow-up of 35 patients. *Acta Orthop Scand* 1993;64:33–36.

Leahy AL, Fogarty EE, Fitzgerald RJ, Regan BF. Discitis as a cause of abdominal pain in children. *Surgery* 1984;95:412–414.

Medical Research Council, War Memorandum No. 7. *Aids to the investigation of peripheral nerve injuries,* 2nd ed. London: His Majesty's Stationery Office, 1943.

Norman MG, McGillvary BC, Kalouselo DK, et al. *Congenital malformations of the brain.* New York: Oxford University Press, 1995.

Smith HP, Hendrick EB. Subdural empyema and epidural abscess in children. *J Neurosurg* 1983;58:392–397.

Chapter 7

Spinal Cord Disease

Case

A 10-year-old girl has a 1-week history of sharp back pain radiating around the left costal margin that is worse with coughing. For the past day, she has had urinary incontinence, and, over the past 5 hours, she has become weak in her legs. Intravenous Decadron is given, and emergency magnetic resonance imaging (MRI) of the spine shows an epidural mass at T-6, with cord compression. She is started on radiation therapy that night, and, over 2 weeks, she gradually improves to baseline.

Diagnosis

Acute spinal cord compression at T-6 that is caused by an epidural bony metastasis from Ewing sarcoma.

Acute spinal cord compression is a neurologic emergency. The prognosis is related to the delay between the onset of neurologic symptoms and treatment. Being alert to the possibility of cord compression is crucial for early diagnosis.

CHARACTERISTIC SYMPTOMS

- Back pain
- Root pain, often radiating around the side or down a limb
- Paresthesias in leg (e.g., "funny feelings," tingling, or numbness)
- Change in urine function (patient urinates more or less frequently)

- Weakness in the lower extremities, especially when climbing stairs
- Constipation or fecal incontinence

Early Signs

- Loss of pinprick sensation or a different reaction to pinprick is seen in the lower extremities. The patient may have a sensory "level" to pinprick. A temperature "level" to a cool object or a "sweat" level may be present.
- Position or vibration loss occurs in the feet.
- Tenderness over the spine is a helpful sign in determining the level of the lesion.
- Slight hyperreflexia in the lower extremities is seen, compared with the upper extremities.

(*Note:* The toes are often down-going, and reflexes may be reduced in early acute cord compression because of spinal shock.)

Late Signs

- Definite weakness
- Definite hyperreflexia
- Up-going toes
- A sensory level to pinprick, temperature, or vibration; often helpful to check vibration sense up and down the spine in search of a level; check for a sweat level
- Loss of anal sphincter tone and voluntary contraction; absent abdominal reflexes, absent bulbocavernosus reflex
- Urinary retention or incontinence of the bowel or bladder

CAUSES OF SPINAL CORD COMPRESSION

Epidural Compression

- Metastatic tumor (neuroblastoma, reticulum cell sarcoma); spinal cord compression may be the initial manifestation of malignancy
- Trauma
- Lymphoma
- Multiple myeloma
- Epidural abscess or hematoma
- Cervical or thoracic disk protrusion or spondylosis or spondylolisthesis
- Atlantoaxial subluxation (trisomy 21)

Extramedullary Intradural Compression

- Meningioma
- Neurofibroma

Intramedullary Expansion

- Glioma
- Ependymoma
- Arteriovenous malformation

DIAGNOSTIC STEPS

- Perform a careful neurologic examination; estimate the level of the cord lesion. Note that the lesion may lie above the sensory level because of partial injury and lamination of sensory tracts. Also note that the dermatomal level does not correspond to the bony level because of the termination of the cord at lower L-2 and upper L-3.
- Check for the site of primary tumor.
- Plain films of the spine may reveal a vertebral collapse or subluxation, bony erosion secondary to tumor, or calcification (meningioma).
- Early consultation with a neurologist or neurosurgeon and a radiation therapist is needed.
- Do not perform a lumbar puncture if cord compression is suspected; imaging the lesion is the initial key to diagnosis and treatment.
- Image the entire spine because multiple sites of compression may be present.

TREATMENT

Treatment depends on the site(s) of cord injury and the etiology. Treatment is most effective if it is instituted early. Acute bowel and bladder dysfunction in the setting of cord compression is an emergency, as is rapidly progressive weakness. Modalities include radiotherapy (reticulum cell sarcoma, lymphoma), surgical decompression for solitary radioresistant extradural solid tumors, or a combination of both. Dexamethasone (12 mg per m^2) is usually given immediately because this may help preserve spinal cord function.

DIFFERENTIAL DIAGNOSIS OF NONCOMPRESSIVE SPINAL CORD INJURY

- **Transverse myelitis** is characterized by the acute or subacute development of paraplegia or quadriplegia—occasionally asymmetric—associated with back pain and sensory loss. It may be related to a preceding viral illness (e.g., infectious mononucleosis). The cerebrospinal fluid may show pleocytosis with increased protein and normal sugar levels. Studies for disorders such as Lyme disease, lupus erythematosus, syphilis, human immunodeficiency virus, cytomegalovirus, herpes simplex virus, and Epstein-Barr virus should be considered. MRI or computed tomography is usually necessary to rule out a compressive lesion. In addition, an MRI may show intramedullary pathology, such as demyelinating disease or intramedullary tumor. Treatment is supportive. Corticosteroids are often used when the etiology is thought to be postinfectious or demyelinating.
- **Radiation myelopathy** usually occurs 6 months to 5 years after irradiation to the thoracic area of the spinal cord. The onset may be insidious or abrupt, and it may be limited to paresthesias or it may progress to actual paralysis. Myelography may be secondary to vascular damage to the spinal cord. Steroids have been used with limited results.
- **Acute spinal cord trauma** is treated with stabilization of the spine and with high dose steroids.
- **Spinal cord injury without observable radiologic abnormalities (SCIWORA).**
  - Traumatic spine injury may be seen.
  - This is usually cervical.
  - The injury can be thoracic.
  - The risk is greater with atlantoaxial instability (i.e., Down syndrome), Chiari malformation, and small canal.
  - Children younger than the age of 8 years are the most susceptible.
  - Elastic biomechanics of pediatric vertebral column allow deformation of spine beyond the usual physiologic limits.
  - Defects result from excessive hyperextension, flexion, and ischemic injury.
  - Plain films and computed tomography may be negative.
  - MRI may be normal, or it may show edema or hemorrhage on both T-1 and T-2.

- The prognosis is poor, and it relates to extent of clinical involvement at time of incident.

Suggested Reading

Dickman CA, Zabramski JM, Hadley MN, et al. Pediatric spinal cord injury without radiographic abnormalities: report of 26 cases and review of the literature. *J Spinal Dis* 1991;4:296–305.

Epstein JA, Lavine LS. Herniated lumbar intervertebral disks in teenage children. *J Neurosurg* 1964;21:1070–1075.

Greenwald TA, Mann DC. Pediatric seatbelt injuries: diagnosis and treatment of lumbar flexion-distraction injuries. *Paraplegia* 1994;32:743–751.

Hadley MN, Zabramski JM, Browner CM, et al. Pediatric spinal trauma. Review of 122 cases of spinal cord and vertebral column injuries. *J Neurosurg* 1988;68:18–24.

Hamilton MG, Myles ST. Pediatric spinal injury: review of 174 hospital admissions. *J Neurosurg* 1992;77:700–704.

Kriss VM, Kriss TC. SCIWORA (Spinal cord injury without radiographic abnormality) in infants and children. *Clin Pediatr* 1996;35:119–124.

Quencer RM, Nunez D, Green BA. Controversies in imaging acute cervical spine trauma. *Am J Neuroradiol* 1997;18:1866–1868.

Ruge JR, Sinson GP, McLone DG, Cerullo LJ. Pediatric spinal injury: the very young. *J Neurosurg* 1988;68:25–30.

Tator CH, Fehlings MG. Review of the secondary injury theory of acute spinal cord trauma with emphasis on vascular mechanisms. *J Neurosurg* 1991;75:15–26.

Chapter 8

Neuropathies

Case

A 1-day-old infant, following breech delivery with associated shoulder dystocia, is found to have an adducted internally rotated arm; the elbow is extended, and the forearm is pronated. Suggested weakness of the deltoid biceps and brachioradialis is seen.

Diagnosis

Erb palsy (upper trunk lesion)
The child recovered over a period of 2 to 3 months.

The peripheral nervous system consists of the 12 cranial nerves originating at the base of the brain and the peripheral nerves derived from the various roots, the plexus, and the trunks of nerves originating from the spinal cord. Disorders of the autonomic nervous system arise from abnormalities of either the sympathetic or parasympathetic system. In childhood, diseases of the autonomic nervous system are distinctly rare.

Disorders of the peripheral nervous system can be either sensory or motor or sensory motor. Diseases of the peripheral nerves may be demyelinating or axonal. As a general rule, demyelinating diseases tend to be less severe and have a much better prognosis for recovery than does axonal disease.

Electromyography (EMG) is much more helpful in the diagnosis of nerve disease than it is in muscle disease. EMG can reliably diagnose whether a process is myopathic, neuropathic, demyelinating, or axonal. Measurement of conduction time and/or compound motor nerve potentials defines whether the process is demyelinating or axonal. Localization of the root involved can also be assessed electromyographically. Most diseases of the peripheral nervous system can be categorized as acute or chronic (Table 8.1).

BIRTH-RELATED BRACHIAL PLEXUS INJURIES

These are commonly thought to be traumatic. However, an increasing body of literature suggests that brachial plexus injury in the newborn may occur without definitive evidence of trauma.

Etiology

- Breech delivery
- Shoulder dystocia
- Excessive traction of the head and shoulder during delivery
- Idiopathic

Clinical Features

- Erb palsy: upper trunk involvement of C-5 and C-6 roots
  - Arm is adducted, internally rotated, elbow extended, and the forearm pronated.
  - Weakness of the deltoid, biceps, and brachioradialis muscles may be present.

TABLE 8.1 Electromyography and Nerve Conduction

	Normal	Muscle	Nerve
Insertional activity	Minimal	Increased	Minimal
Fibrillation	Absent	Absent to minimal	Increased
Compound motor action potential	Normal	Decreased, short duration	Increased, long duration
Positive sharp waves	Absent	Absent to increased	Increased
Recruitment	Readily elicited	Increased	Decreased
Nerve conduction velocity	Normal	Normal	Decreased

- ◆ Extension of the arm is limited.
- ◆ Fingers may be fisted.
- ◆ Biceps and triceps reflexes are lost.

- Klumpke: lower trunk involvement of the C-8 and T-1 roots
  - ◆ Horner syndrome (meiosis, ptosis, and anhidrosis) is found.
  - ◆ Elbow is flexed.
  - ◆ Forearm is supinated.
  - ◆ Wrist is extended.
  - ◆ Hand is claw-like.
  - ◆ Forearm extensors, flexion of the wrist and fingers, and intrinsic muscles of the hand are weak.
- Complete brachial plexus injury
  - ◆ Hand hangs limply at the side
  - ◆ Absent reflexes
  - ◆ No evident movement of the limb

Treatment

- Pin arm in sling to prevent further injury when sleeping.
- Initiate passive range of motion exercises to maintain and prevent contractures.
- Seventy percent to 80% make full recovery. Recovery may take weeks to months.
- In the absence of improvement after 2 to 3 months, consider reanastomosis of nerves.

BRACHIAL PLEXITIS

- Symptoms begin with pain in the neck or shoulder.
- Decreased deep tendon reflexes are seen.
- Long thoracic nerve with scapular winging is involved.
- This may be inherited in an autosomal dominant manner linked to chromosome 17q
- The initial recovery is usually complete, but exacerbations may be associated with residual weakness.

INFLAMMATORY DEMYELINATING POLYRADICULOPATHY (GUILLAIN-BARRÉ SYNDROME)

- Acute or subacute
- May have proximal muscle weakness

- Thought to be initiated by infection, which triggers an autoimmune response
- Commonly identified infectious agents
  - *Campylobacter jejunum*
  - Epstein-Barr virus
  - Mumps

Clinical Features

- Disease may begin days to weeks after an infection.
- Symptoms may begin with pain in the thighs and difficulty in getting up off the floor and/or difficulty climbing up and down stairs.
- Symmetric weakness initially involves the lower extremities; proximal weakness is usually greater than distal.
- Reflexes are absent early in the course of the disease.
- Disease may progress rapidly over 24 to 72 hours with complete bulbar paralysis and respiratory compromise.
- Autonomic involvement may be associated with hypertension, blurred vision, and cardiac arrhythmias.
- Bladder and bowel incontinence is rare—urinary retention is seen in up to 25% of patients.
- Papilledema is rare.

Electromyography and Nerve Conduction

- Decreased nerve conduction
- Decreased compound motor action potentials (suggests axonal involvement)
- Decreased to absent F waves

Lumbar Puncture

- Albuminocytologic association: increased protein in the absence of cells

Treatment

- Intravenous immune globulin (probably the treatment of choice)—0.4 g per kg per day for 5 days or 2 g per kg per day for 2 days
- Plasmapheresis
- Early ventilatory support, especially if vital capacities or peak flows are trending downward

Prognosis

Most recover without sequelae.

CHRONIC INFLAMMATORY POLYNEUROPATHY

- Clinical presentation similar to Guillain-Barré syndrome
- Immune-mediated polyneuropathy of greater than 2 months' duration
- Albuminocytologic disassociation
- May relapse

Electromyography and Nerve Conduction

- Decreased nerve conduction velocity
- Decreased or absent F waves
- Conduction block

Treatment

- Dramatic response to steroids
- Intravenous immune globulin or plasmapheresis if refractory to steroids

HEREDITARY SENSORY NEUROPATHIES

Characteristics

- May be dominant, recessive, or sex linked, depending on family pedigree
- Seven types as follows:
  - Charcot-Marie Tooth, type I
  - Charcot-Marie Tooth, type II
  - Dejerine-Sottas disease: hypomyelinating neuropathies, type III
  - Refsum disease, type IV
  - Sensory motor neuropathy with pyramidal features, type V
  - Sensory motor neuropathy with optic atrophy, type VI
  - Sensory motor neuropathy with retinitis pigmentosa, type VII

Clinical Features

- Peroneal muscular atrophy
- Champagne bottle or stork-like legs

- Foot drop
- Pes cavus
- Sensory loss
- Areflexia
- May be associated, depending on type, with optic atrophy, retinitis pigmentosa, and/or cerebellar and pyramidal signs
- Kyphosis and scoliosis in approximately 10%

Course

- Usually progressive throughout adolescence and early adulthood, then plateaus
- Many different presentations depending on family pedigree
- May have associated upper extremity findings
- Variable cerebellar findings
- Compatible with long life with significant disability

Treatment

- Ankle foot orthoses
- Orthopedic surgery
- Physical and occupational therapies

NEUROPATHIES DIAGNOSED BY PATHOLOGY

Giant Axonal Neuropathy

- Kinky hair
- Long curly eyelashes
- Mental retardation
- Spasticity
- Sensory motor neuropathy
- Pathology—swollen axons with densely packed neurofilaments

Infantile Neuroaxonal Dystrophy

- Onset at 1 to 2 years of age
- Mental retardation
- Seizures
- Decreased deep tendon reflexes
- Mineralization of the basal ganglion
- Sensory motor neuropathy
- Autonomic neuropathy

- Pathology—central peripheral and autonomic neurons contain spheroids of varying size
- Ballooned axons positive for Periodic–acid Schiff reaction

SYSTEMIC NEUROPATHIES

- Diabetes
- Uremia
- Porphyria
- Vitamin deficiencies
- Heavy metal—lead, arsenic, and mercury
- Chemotherapy—platinum, vincristine, paclitaxel, and thalidomide
- Toxic neuropathies—diptheria and botulism

COMPRESSION NEUROPATHIES

Brachial Plexus Injuries

- Associated with fracture of the clavicle
- Also seen with dislocation of the humerus
- Upper plexus more commonly affected than the lower plexus
- Recovery: proximal to distal

Lumbar Plexus Injuries

Seen with fracture of the pelvis.

Median Neuropathy (C6 to T1) (Fig. 8.1)

- Compression in the carpal tunnel
- Muscles involved as follows:
  - Thumb flexion, abduction and opposition
  - Flexion of the index and middle finger, proximal joint flexion, distal interphalangeal extension
  - Sensory loss in the thumb and first two fingers, the palmar surface of hand, the distal interphalangeal joints, and dorsal surface of hand
- Pain in the hand with sparing of the ulnar half of the fourth and fifth fingers
- Tinel sign at the wrist when the carpal tunnel is involved
- May also occur with trauma to the axilla or elbow

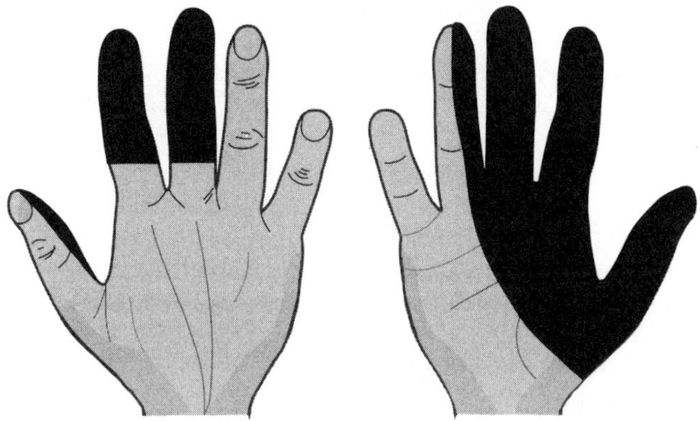

FIGURE 8.1 Median sensory loss. (From Weiner HL, Levitt LP, Rae-Grant A. *Neurology*, 6th ed. Philadelphia: Lippincott Williams & Wilkins, 1999, with permission.)

Ulnar Neuropathy (C8 to T1) (Fig. 8.2)

- External pressure or subluxation of the nerve in the olecranon groove
- Traumatic injury at the elbow
- Following muscles involved:
  - Ulnar flexion at wrist
  - Ring and fifth finger flexion
  - Interossei and fourth and fifth lumbricals

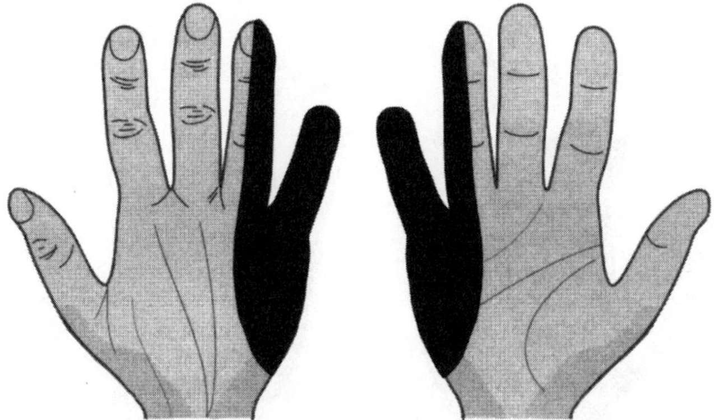

FIGURE 8.2 Ulnar sensory loss. (From Weiner HL, Levitt LP, Rae-Grant A. *Neurology*, 6th ed. Philadelphia: Lippincott Williams & Wilkins, 1999, with permission.)

- Fracture of the distal humerus
- Paresthesias of the ulnar side of the hand
- Weakness of the intrinsic muscles of the hand
- Sensory loss in fourth and little finger and medial side of hand
- Claw hand
- May also involve associated Horner syndrome

Radial neuropathy (C5 to C8) (Fig. 8.3)

- Injury to the nerve occurs either in the axilla or radial groove of the humerus below the take-off of the branch to the triceps
- Pressure injury or fracture of the humerus
- Muscles involved as follows:
  - Supinator
  - Extensor of the upper arm, forearm, and fingers
- Wrist drop—most common injury
- Sensory loss on the dorsal lateral side of hand

Peroneal Neuropathy

- Compression at the lateral edge of the fibula as it leaves the tibial nerve in the popliteal fossa—nerve divides into the superficial and deep peroneal nerves
- Acute painless foot drop
- Muscles involved as follows:
  - Anterior tibialis, dorsiflexion of the foot
  - Peroneal longus and brevis, foot evertors

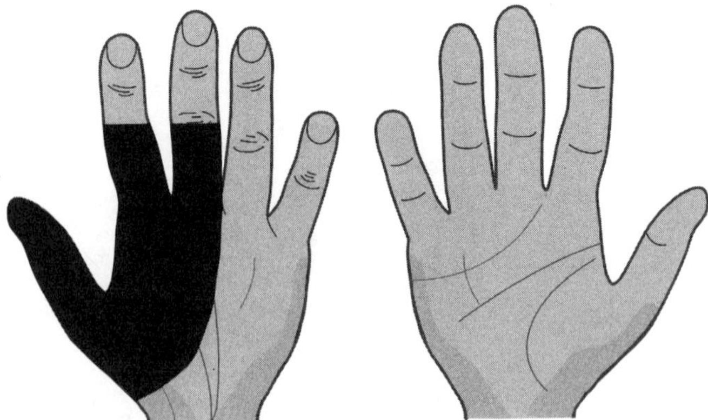

FIGURE 8.3 Radial sensory loss. (From Weiner HL, Levitt LP, Rae-Grant A. *Neurology*, 6th ed. Philadelphia: Lippincott Williams & Wilkins, 1999, with permission.)

- Weakness of dorsiflexion of the foot
- Decreased sensation of the dorsum of the foot and the lateral aspect of the leg

BELL PALSY: ACUTE FACIAL NEUROPATHY (CRANIAL NERVE VII) OF IDIOPATHIC ORIGIN

Clinical Features

Lower motor seventh neuropathy, either partial or complete, with the following features:

- Inability to close the eyes
- Inability to purse lips
- Inability to close mouth fully
- Loss of nasolabial fold
- Loss of ability to wrinkle forehead
- Drooling
- Tearing of the eyes
- Hyperacusis

Anatomy

- Involvement of the seventh nerve anywhere between the seventh nerve nucleus in the pons, the internal auditory meatus, the middle ear, and its exit at the stylomastoid foramen (Fig. 8.4).
- May involve any branch of the seventh nerve.
  - Temporal
  - Zygomatic
  - Buccal
  - Mandibular
  - Cervical

Course

- Usually benign
- Resolves in 2 weeks to 6 months
- EMG not prognostic before 14 days to 3 weeks
- Any movement of facial muscle suggests complete recovery
- Steroids rarely helpful

Consider Bell Palsy if No Etiology Found

Some Possible Etiologies

- Herpes zoster (involvement of the geniculate ganglion)
- Guillain-Barré syndrome

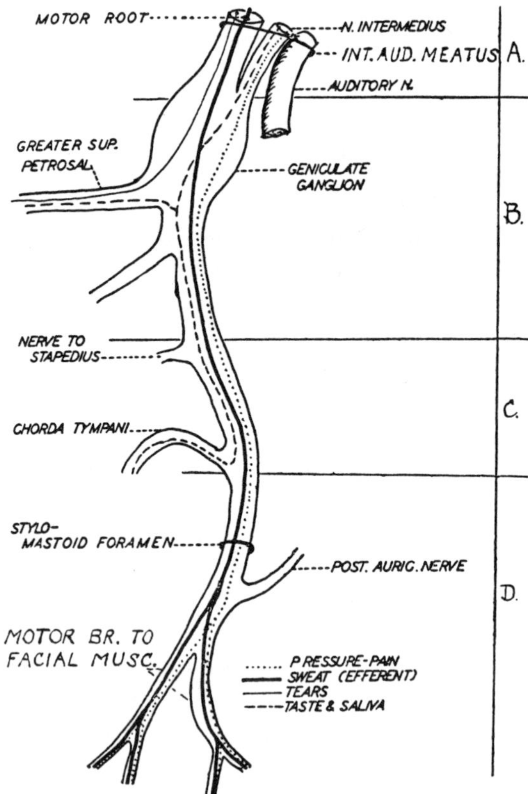

FIGURE 8.4 Diagram illustrating the course of the various parts of the facial nerve. **A:** Proximal part of facial nerve between the internal auditory meatus and the geniculate ganglion. **B:** Ganglionic part of facial nerve and trunk up to a point proximal to the origin of the nerve to the stapedius. **C:** Trunk of the facial nerve up to and including the origin of chorda tympani branch. **D:** Distal part of the facial nerve. (From Brock S, Kreiger HP. *Basis of clinical neurology.* Baltimore: Williams & Wilkins, 1963, with permission.)

- Myasthenia gravis
- Trauma
- Brainstem glioma
- Lupus
- Leukemia

- Melkersson syndrome
- Epstein-Barr infection
- Mycoplasma infection
- Lyme disease

Suggested Reading

Adler JB, Patterson RL. Erb's palsy: long term results of treatment in eighty-eight cases. *J Bone Joint Surg Am* 1967;49:1052–1064.

Bradshaw DY, Jones HR Jr. Guillain-Barré syndrome in children: clinical course, electrodiagnosis, and prognosis. *Muscle Nerve* 1992;15:500–506.

Dyck PJ, Thomas PK, Griffin JW, et al., eds. *Peripheral neuropathy*. Philadelphia: WB Saunders, 1993.

Eng GD. Brachial plexus palsy in newborn infants. *Pediatrics* 1971;48:18–28.

Eng GD, Binder H, Getson P, O'Donnell R. Obstetrical brachial plexus palsy (OBPP) outcome with conservative management. *Muscle Nerve* 1996;19:884–891.

Epstein MA, Sladky JT. The role of plasmapheresis in childhood Guillain-Barré syndrome. *Ann Neurol* 1990;28:65–69.

Fenichel GM. *Clinical pediatric neurology: a signs and symptoms approach,* 4th ed. Philadelphia: WB Saunders, 2001.

Greenwald AG, Schute PC, Shiveley JL. Brachial plexus birth palsy: a 10-year report on the incidence and prognosis. *J Pediatr Orthop* 1984;4:689–692.

Hagberg B, Lyon G. Pooled European series of hereditary peripheral neuropathies in infancy and childhood. *Neuropaediatrie* 1981;12:9–17.

Lamont PJ, Johnston HM, Berdoukas VA. Plasmapheresis in children with Guillain-Barré syndrome. *Neurology* 1991;41:1928–1931.

Langworth EP, Taverner D. The prognosis in facial palsy. *Brain* 1963;86:465.

Nordborg C, Conradi N, Sourander P, et al. Hereditary motor and sensory neuropathy of demyelinating and remyelinating type in children: ultrastructural and morphometric studies on sural nerve biopsy specimens from ten sporadic cases. *Acta Neuropathol* 1984;64:1–9.

Ouvrier R, McLeod JG, Pollard J. *Peripheral neuropathy in childhood.* New York: Raven Press, 1990. International Review of Child Neurology Series.

Plasmapheresis and acute Guillain-Barré syndrome. The Guillain-Barré syndrome study group. *Neurology* 1985;35:1096–1104.

Ropper AH, Wijdick, Elco FM, et al. The Guillain-Barré syndrome. In: *Contemporary Neurology Series.* Philadelphia: FA Davis, 1991.

Wiederholt WC. Hereditary brachial neuropathy: report of two families. *Arch Neurol* 1974;30:252–254.

Wolf SM, Wagner JH Jr, Davidson S, et al. Treatment of Bell palsy with prednisone: a prospective randomized study. *Neurology* 1978;28:158–161.

Chapter 9

Muscle Diseases

Case

A 3-week-old infant is seen in the newborn nursery. She has a history of decreased tone and failure to suck, and she has a long, narrow facies. A biopsy shows rod-like elements scattered throughout most of the muscle.

Diagnosis

Nemaline rod myopathy
The family is told that the child may get slightly better with age but that she will continue to have significant muscle weakness.

CONGENITAL MYOPATHIES

Congenital myopathies represent developmental, rather than destructive, disease of the muscle. Because they do not involve destruction of muscle, the course is characterized by a slight improvement with age, stability, or an extremely slow progression. These entities are commonly considered in the diagnosis of a floppy infant. Weakness, as in spinal muscular atrophy, is noted either at birth or in the first several months of life. It is generally proximal, with the preservation of reflexes. Creatine phosphokinase (CPK) is usually normal, or it may be modestly elevated. The diagnosis is primarily made by muscle biopsy. Electromyography (EMG) offers little or no help, and, at times, it can be confusing. Although some congenital myopathies, like nemaline rod, may have suggestive phenotypic features, the diagnosis is usually considered on clinical examination and is definitively made by muscle biopsy. Several congenital myopathies are described below.

Central Core Disease

- Condition is autosomal dominant.
- Gene locus is on chromosome 19q13. May be allelic for malignant hyperthermia.
- Patients present as floppy infants with proximal weakness.
- Pathology reveals centrally placed cores of degenerative myofibrils in the center of type 1 fibers.
- Central cores are best demonstrated using oxidative enzymes (nicotinamide adenine dinucleotide [NADH]-tetrazolium reductase reaction).

Congenital Fiber Type Disproportion

- Inheritance is variable.
- Patient usually presents as a floppy infant.
- Joint contractures, hip dislocation, and/or arthrogryposis may be part of the clinical syndrome.
- Historically, type 1 predominance and hypotrophy are seen.

Myotubular Myopathy

- Inheritance is variable; it can be X-linked or mendelian.
- Proximal weakness is seen in infancy.
- Respiratory difficulties may be seen.
- Pathology is type 1 fiber prominence and hypotrophy.
- Muscle biopsy shows internal nuclei with increased evidence of oxidative enzymes.

Nemaline (Rod Body) Myopathy

- Proximal weakness
- Floppy infant
- Myopathic facies, long and narrow
- Club feet
- Kyphoscoliosis
- Rod-like elements on biopsy—scattered throughout most of the muscle fibers, type 1 fiber predominance
- Variable course, usually benign

MUSCULAR DYSTROPHIES

The muscular dystrophies, unlike the congenital myopathies, are characterized by the progressive destruction of muscle. As a result, most children become worse over time. Muscle enzymes may be elevated, and EMGs are more likely to be diagnostic of a myopathy.

Congenital Muscular Dystrophy

- This condition is present at birth or soon thereafter.
- Abnormality of merosin and linking protein in skeletal muscle is seen; this can also be expressed in the cerebrospinal fluid.
- Gene abnormality is on chromosome 6q2.
- Inheritance can be either dominant or recessive.
- Magnetic resonance imaging shows a marked increase in T-2 signals in the white matter; these increase over time.
- Muscle biopsy suggests a dystrophic process with degeneration of muscle, fatty, and collagen replacement and little evidence of regeneration.

Fukuyama Type C and D

- Cerebral dysplasia with muscular dystrophy is seen.
- Gene is located on chromosome 9q31-33.
- Polymicrogyria, lissencephaly, and heterotropias are common.
- Contractures may be present at birth.
- Mental retardation can be severe.
- Microcephaly is common.
- Weakness may be proximal or distal.
- Muscle biopsy shows degeneration of muscle with replacement of fat and collagen tissue.

Duchenne and Becker Type

- Duchenne presents at 2 to 4 years of age. Becker presents late in childhood, or it may be delayed until adolescence.
- The early symptoms are delayed walking, a waddling gait, difficulty running, and increased shuffling.
- CPK may be elevated before the onset of clinical signs.
- Patients have difficulty arising from the floor and chair; they push off with their hands and climb up their legs (Gower sign).
- Calf hypertrophy is seen.

- Gene locus is on Xp21.
- Disease is X-linked recessive.
- Gene product is reduced with loss of muscle content of dystrophin.
- In Duchenne dystrophy, the dystrophin content is less than 3% of normal, whereas, in Becker dystrophy, the dystrophin content can be up to 20% of normal.
- Onset and weakness in Becker dystrophy occur later than in Duchenne dystrophy, and the course is not malignant.
- The course of Duchenne is invariably progressive, with loss of ambulation and/or death in late adolescence or early adulthood.
- Respiratory failure and/or cardiomyopathy occur late in the disease.
- Some evidence suggests that daily prednisone may delay the symptoms.

FASCIOSCAPULOHUMERAL DYSTROPHY (FOLLICLE-STIMULATING HORMONE)

- Although this is thought to be primarily a muscle disease, patterns of follicle-stimulating hormone (FSH) may be seen in certain neuropathies.
- Gene is located on 4q35.
- This usually occurs in the second decade; it starts in the shoulder girdle with subsequent involvement of the face.
- The lower extremities may also be involved.
- Proximal weakness is in the arms, and distal weakness is in the legs. Without involvement of the face, this suggests scapuloperoneal syndrome.
- CPK may be normal or increased.
- EMG may be confusing, showing both neuropathic and myopathic potentials.
- The course is variable; little or no disability may be seen, or the course may be characterized by a more progressive nature.

LIMB GIRDLE DYSTROPHY

- Progressive and symmetric weakness is seen, with sparing of the face.
- The condition is autosomal recessive.
- It is usually benign in adolescence and early adulthood.
- The defect is in adhalin, which is part of the dystrophin–glycoprotein complex.

- The EMG suggests myopathy
- The biopsy confirms myopathic pattern.

MYOTONIC DYSTROPHY

Genetics (Table 9.1)

- Autosomal dominant
- Gene incidence: 1 in 80,000
- Three genotypes
  - Type 1: CTG expansion in the noncoding region on chromosome 19
  - Congenital myotonic dystrophy: same as Type 1
  - Type 2: CTG expansion in noncoding region on chromosome 3; recent information suggests that this condition is due to a tetranucleotide repeat of CCTG rather than to the trinucleotide repeat of CTG

Clinical Characteristics

- Myotonia: increased contraction, followed by delayed relaxation of the affected muscles
- Elicited by percussion of the thenar eminence, tongue, or deltoid muscles
- Symptoms enhanced by cold

Electromyogram

- Spontaneous discharges on needle insertion
- Characteristic "dive bomber sound"

Clinical Features

- Classic
  - Proximal weakness
  - Facial diplegia
  - Ptosis
  - Cataracts
  - Frontal balding
  - Ophthalmoplegia
  - Cardiac conduction defects
  - Diabetes
  - Mother affected with myotonic dystrophy more likely to have affected child than is an affected father

- Mild form—similar to classic form except much milder with limited muscle involvement

Congenital Myotonic Dystrophy

- Respiratory feeding difficulties at birth
- Inverted "V" or tented "T" sign (i.e., inability to approximate lip closure)
- Talipes equinovarus
- Improvement in strength over time
- Fifty percent to 60% retarded
- Myotonia not present at birth; develops in early to late childhood
- Predisposition to malignant hyperthermia with anesthesia

PERIODIC PARALYSIS

Hyperkalemic Periodic Paralysis

- Autosomal dominant, chromosome 17
- Channelopathy
- Age at onset: first decade
- Cold, rest, and potassium provoke symptoms
- Potassium elevated during attack
- Responds to thiazides, acetazolamide
- Responds to sodium restriction

Hypokalemic Periodic Paralysis

- Autosomal dominant, chromosome 1
- Affects alpha I subunit of calcium channel
- First or second decade
- Provocative symptoms: rest, high carbohydrate diet, cold
- Decreased potassium during the attack; at low normal or below normal
- Responds to oral potassium, acetazolamide, spironolactone, and low sodium and low carbohydrate diet

Juvenile Dermatomyositis

This systemic angiopathy is characterized by small vessel vasculitis. The diagnosis is made if four of the following symptoms are found:

- Muscle weakness
- Elevated CPK

TABLE 9.1 Relationship of CTG Repeats to Clinical Phenotype of Myotonic Dystrophy

Phenotype	Repeat Size	Age at Onset (yr)
Premutation	35–49	Normal
Mild	50–150	20–70
Classic	100–1,500	10–30
Congenital[a]	100–1,500	10–30

[a] Congenital form is associated with anticipation; in other words, the greater the number of repeats, the more likely the disease is to be severe. In affected individuals, the contributing parent, usually the mother, may have a limited number of repeats and mild disease, whereas the offspring with increased repeats develops the congenital form.

- Fibrillation on EMG
- Cutaneous rash
- Fascicular atrophy and mononuclear perivascular infiltrates on muscle biopsy

Peak incidence is at 5 to 10 years of age.

Clinical

- May present acutely (30%) or insidiously with prodrome of fever, fatigue, weight loss, muscle weakness
- Painful and tender muscles
- Muscle stiffness
- Proximal and symmetric muscle weakness
  - Difficulty climbing stairs, brushing hair
  - Positive Gower sign (difficulty getting from a supine to standing position; child "climbs up" his or her legs, using arms to stand)
  - Neck flexor weakness seen early
- Contractures seen early
- Bulbar muscles: dysphagia seen in approximately one-third of patients

Skin Findings

These often precede muscle symptoms.

- Heliotrope rash
  - Violaceous hue on eyelids spreading to periorbital and malar regions
  - Periorbital edema

- Gottron papules—erythematous papular lesions with induration; progresses to atrophy of the dorsum metacarpophalangeal and interphalangeal joints of hands. May also involve the extensor surfaces of the knees and elbows.
- Maculopapular scaly rash
  - Diffuse
  - Upper torso and extensor surfaces
- Skin vasculitis
  - "Splinter hemorrhages" nailbeds—seen best after putting immersion oil on the nailbeds and observing with an ophthalmoscope at +15 to +40.
  - May develop ulceration of the skin, fingers, and oral mucosa
- Calcinosis (subcutaneous) in 30% to 70%; may erupt through the skin
- Generalized disease
  - Myocarditis and/or pericarditis, arrhythmia, and conduction defects
  - Pneumonic infiltrates (rare), interstitial lung disease
  - Vasculitis bowel, leading to gastrointestinal infarction and ulceration
    - May be fatal
    - Can cause malabsorption, ulcers, perforation, hemorrhage
  - Renal involvement—hematuria, proteinuria; rare
  - Cerebritis
  - Calcinosis of the subcutaneous tissue (50% of children)
  - No increased incidence of cancer (unlike the disease seen in adults)

Evaluation

- Muscle enzymes
  - Increased CPK (90%), aldolase, and aspartate aminotransferase
  - Creatine kinase may not correlate with weakness
- Increased Factor VIII—reflects the activity of vasculitis
- Serum complement—may have decreased C-4 and C-3
- Increased antinuclear antibodies (ANA)—25% to 50% of patients
- Lymphopenia
- Erythrocyte sedimentation rate—normal or elevated
- EMG

- Not specific
- Increased insertional activity
- Positive sharp waves at rest
- Small amplitude
- Fibrillation
- Polyphasic potentials on contraction

- Muscle biopsy
  - Perifascicular atrophy (90%)
  - Perivascular lymphocytic infiltrates
  - Involves small arterioles, capillaries, and small venules
- Computed tomography and x-ray—may show calcinosis

Treatment

Early aggressive treatment limits contractures and calcinosis.

- Limit activity during the acute phase
- When inflammation goes down, begin intensive physical therapy to prevent contractures
- Steroids
  - Prednisone, 2 mg per kg per day, divided into 4 doses (maximum dose, 100 mg/day). High dose for several months, then switch to alternate day regimen. Treat for 2 years. **OR**
  - Methylprednisolone, 30 mg per kg per day, up to 1 g intravenously every 24 to 48 hours until inflammation subsides. Then, switch to oral corticosteroids.
- If response to steroids is poor, try the following:
  - Methotrexate, 10 mg per m^2 per wk
  - Intravenous immune globulin, 2 g per kg, over 2 to 5 days
  - Hydroxychloroquine for dermatitis: repeat every 2 to 6 weeks for 3 months minimum. Proven efficacy in adults with dermatomyositis.
- Plasmapheresis: ineffective in controlled trial

Outcome

The outcome is variable. It may resolve or it can become chronic.

Suggested Reading

Baumbach LL, Chamberlain JS, Ward PS, et al. Molecular and clinical correlations of deletions leading to Duchenne and Becker muscular dystrophies. *Neurology* 1989;39:465–475.

Berkovic SF, Carpenter S, Evans A, et al. Myoclonus epilepsy and ragged-red fibers (MERRF). 1. A clinical, pathological, biochemical, magnetic resonance spectrographic and positron emission tomography study. *Brain* 1989;112:1231–1260.

Brook JD, McCurrach ME, Harley HG, et al. Molecular basis of myotonic dystrophy: expansion of a trinucleotide (CTG) repeat at the 3′ end of a transcript encoding a protein kinase family member. *Cell* 1992;68: 799–808.

Brown MD, Wallace DC. Molecular basis of mitochondrial DNA disease. *J Bioenerg Biomembr* 1994;26:273–289.

Cannon SC. From mutation to myotonia in sodium channel disorders. *Neuromusc Disord* 1997;7:241–249.

Cannon SC. Sodium channel defects in myotonia and periodic paralysis. *Annu Rev Neurosci* 1996;19:141–164.

Cook JD, Gascon GG, Haider A, et al. Congenital muscular dystrophy with abnormal radiographic myelin pattern. *J Child Neurol* 1992;7: S51–S63.

DiMauro S. Mitochondrial encephalomyopathies. In: Rosenberg RN, Prusiner SB, DiMauro S, et al, eds. *The molecular and genetic basis of neurological disease.* Boston: Butterworth-Heinemann, 1993.

DiMauro S, Tonin P, Servidei S. Metabolic myopathies. In: Rowland LP, DiMauro S, eds. *Handbook of clinical neurology.* Vol. 18. *Myopathies.* Amsterdam: Elsevier Science Publishers, 1992.

Dubowitz V. *Muscle disorders in childhood,* 2nd ed. London: WB Saunders, 1995.

Fukuyama U, Osawa M, Suzuki H. Congenital progressive muscular dystrophy of the Fukuyama type: clinical, genetic and pathological considerations. *Brain Dev* 1981;3:1–29.

Goebel HH. Congenital myopathies. *Semin Pediatr Neurol* 1996;3:152–161.

Greenberg DA. Calcium channels in neurological disease. *Ann Neurol* 1997;42:275–282.

Griggs RC, Engel WK, Resnick JS. Acetazolamide treatment of hypokalemic periodic paralysis. Prevention of attacks and improvement of persistent weakness. *Ann Intern Med* 1970;73:39–48.

Hoffman EP, Fischbeck MD, Brown RH, et al. Characterization of dystrophin in muscle-biopsy specimens from patients with Duchenne's or Becker's muscular dystrophy. *N Engl J Med* 1988;318:1363–1368.

Huang JL. Long-term prognosis of patients with juvenile dermatomyositis initially treated with intravenous methylprednisolone pulse therapy. *Clin Exp Rheumatol* 1999;17:621–624.

Lapie P, Lory P, Fontaine B. Hypokalemic periodic paralysis: an autosomal dominant muscle disorder caused by mutations in a voltage-gated calcium channel. *Neuromusc Disord* 1997;7:234–240.

Lehmann-Horn F, Rudel R. Channelopathies: the nondystrophic myotonias and periodic paralyses. *Semin Pediatr Neurol* 1996;3:122–139.

Mendell JR, Sahenk Z, Prior TW. The childhood muscular dystrophies: diseases sharing a common pathogenesis of membrane instability. *J Child Neurol* 1995;10:150–159.

North KN, Specht LA, Sethi RK, et al. Congenital muscular dystrophy associated with merosin deficiency. *J Child Neurol* 1996;11:291–295.

O'Neil KM. Juvenile dermatomyositis and polymyositis. In: Finberg L, Kleinman RE, eds. *Saunders manual of pediatric practice,* 2nd ed. Philadelphia: WB Saunders, 2002: 330–333.

Pachman LM. Juvenile dermatomyositis: pathophysiology and disease expression. *Pediatr Clin North Am* 1995;42:1071–1098.

Ptacek LJ, Johnson KG, Griggs RC. Genetics and physiology of the myotonic muscle disorders. *N Engl J Med* 1993;328:482–489.

Robinson BH, DeMeirleir LJ, Glerum M, et al. Clinical presentation of patients with mitochondrial respiratory chain defects in NADH-coenzyme Q reductase and cytochrome oxidase: clues to the pathogenesis of Leigh disease. *J Pediatr* 1987;110:216–222.

Rowland LP. Clinical concepts of Duchenne muscular dystrophy. *Brain* 1988;111:479–495.

Takahashi S, Miyamoto A, Oki J, et al. CTG trinucleotide repeat length and clinical expression in a family with myotonic dystrophy. *Brain Dev* 1996;18:127–130.

Chapter 10

Myasthenia Gravis

Case

A 5-year-old girl is brought to the office with a history of difficulty with swallowing over a period of 4 to 5 weeks. She also has ptosis, and she recently has had some difficulty climbing down and up stairs. The neurologic examination reveals dysarthria, ptosis, and mild proximal weakness. Muscle antibodies sent for acetylcholine receptor antibodies are found to be highly positive. The child has a decremental response on electromyography and a positive response to Tensilon.

Diagnosis

Myasthenia gravis

CLASSIC MYASTHENIA GRAVIS

- Weakness of ocular, bulbar, and striated muscles
- Diplopia
- Difficulty swallowing
- Ptosis
- Proximal muscles more affected than distal
- Weakness increases with the following:
  - Stress
  - Exertion
  - Progression of the day
- Progression to generalized disease in most

- Remains localized (i.e., ocular) in less than 20%
- Respiratory compromise

Associated Disease

- Endocrinopathies (e.g., thyroid)
- Rheumatoid arthritis
- Diabetes
- Systemic lupus erythematosus
- Thymoma (rare in children)

Diagnosis

- Tensilon test (0.1 mg per kg, up to 10 mg)
  - Give test dose of 1 mg
  - Bradycardia and cardiac arrest rare; however, should have atropine available
  - Positive result immediately
- Neostigmine
  - 2 mg per kg orally or 0.04 mg per kg intravenously
  - Positive result in about 15 minutes
- Electromyogram—greater than 10% decremental response of compound muscle action potential with repetitive stimulation
- Antibodies
  - Increased acetylcholine receptor antibodies positive in 80% to 90% of cases of generalized myasthenia
  - Antibodies less likely to be positive in pure ocular myasthenia
  - No correlation of titers with disease severity

Treatment

- Anticholinesterase agents
  - Mestinon
  - Prostigmine
- Thymectomy
  - Consider only when patients are refractory to therapy
  - Results may not be seen for months to years
- Immunosuppressive agents
  - Corticosteroids
    - May be drug of first choice.
    - Initially give prednisone, 2 mg per kg per day. If improvement is seen, slowly wean to every other day.
    - May need to give steroids every other day for 4 to 6 months in conjunction with acetylcholinesterase inhibitors.

    - May worsen the first 7 to 10 days after introduction to steroids. During this time, the patient may need hospitalization.
  - Other immunosuppressive agents
    - Azathioprine
    - Cyclosporine
    - Cyclophosphamide
- Plasmapheresis—remove acetylcholine receptor antibodies
  - Considered first line of treatment in myasthenic crisis
  - Consider in patients with respiratory compromise
  - Consider before and after thymectomy
- Intravenous immunoglobulin—not as well studied as plasmapheresis
  - Indications same as plasmapheresis
  - Response not as dramatic as with plasmapheresis
  - Easy to administer

NEONATAL MYASTHENIA GRAVIS

- Transient
- Seen in approximately 10% of infants of myasthenic mothers
- Represents placental transfer of acetylcholine receptor antibodies
- Presents at birth or in the first 2 to 3 days of life
- Weak suck
- Weak cry
- Dysphasia
- Generalized weakness
- Course usually transient
  - Resolves in 3 to 4 weeks, although occasionally persists for months
  - Treatment with acetylcholinesterase inhibitors usually not necessary

CONGENITAL MYASTHENIA GRAVIS

- Rare—classified into three physiologic categories
  - Presynaptic deficits
  - Synaptic deficits
  - Postsynaptic deficits
- Usually presents within the first 2 years of life
- Probably recessive

- Antibody titers negative
- Does not respond to immunosuppressive therapy
- May respond in limited fashion to acetylcholinesterase inhibitor

Suggested Reading

Anlar B, Ozdirim E, Renda Y, et al. Myasthenia gravis in childhood. *Acta Paediatr* 1996;85:838–842.

Dau PC, Lindstrom JM, Cassel CK, et al. Plasmapheresis and immunosuppressive drug therapy in myasthenia gravis. *N Engl J Med* 1977;297: 1134–1140.

Drachman DB. Myasthenia gravis (first of two parts). *N Engl J Med* 1978; 298:136–142.

Drachman DB. Myasthenia gravis. *N Engl J Med* 1994;330:1797–1810.

Engel AG. Congenital myasthenic syndromes. *Neurol Clin* 1994;12:401–437.

Fenichel GM. Clinical syndrome of myasthenia in infancy and childhood. *Arch Neurol* 1978;35:97–103.

Janas JS, Barohn RJ. A clinical approach to the congenital myasthenic syndromes. *J Child Neurol* 1995;10:168–169.

Misulis KE, Fenichel GM. Genetic forms of myasthenia gravis. *Pediatr Neurol* 1989;5:205–210.

Palace J, Newsom-Davis J, Lecky B, et al. A multicenter, randomized, double-blind trial of prednisolone plus azathioprine versus prednisolone plus placebo in myasthenia gravis. *Neurology* 1996;46:A332.

Shillito P, Vincent A, Newsom-David J. Congenital myasthenic syndromes. *Neuromusc Disord* 1993;3:183–190.

Swaiman KF, Ashwal S. *Pediatric neurology: principles & practice,* 3rd ed. Vol. 2. St. Louis: Mosby, 1999.

Chapter 11

Cerebral Palsy

Case

A 15-month-old infant presented for evaluation of delayed walking. She was the 30-week product of an uncomplicated pregnancy with premature delivery. No problems occurred perinatally. She did not begin sitting until 10 months of age, and she required positioning to prevent her from hyperextending her legs. She was ambidextrous, and she played with small toys. Her receptive and expressive language was appropriate for age. On examination, she was alert and social with an esotropia. She had spasticity in her legs with slight, increased tone in the arms. Her reflexes were increased with clonus and Babinski. When she was put in a standing position, she "scissored" secondary to tightness of her hip adductors. Magnetic resonance imaging revealed periventricular leukomalacia.

Diagnosis

Spastic diplegia (static encephalopathy)

DEFINITION

Cerebral palsy is a static and nonprogressive disorder arising from prenatal or perinatal damage to the motor fibers of the brain with or without associated cognitive defects. The prevalence is 2.5 per 1,000 live births.

RISK FACTORS

Prenatal Events

- Infections: cytomegalovirus, toxoplasmosis, herpes (type I), human immunodeficiency virus
- Pregnancy: third trimester bleeding, alcohol, illicit drugs, polyhydramnios, oligohydramnios, intrauterine growth retardation, maternal epilepsy, maternal mental retardation, maternal hyperthyroidism, toxemia, teenage mother, incompetent cervix

Perinatal Events

- Delivery: precipitous prolonged bleeding, placenta previa or abruptio, premature rupture of membranes, meconium staining, nuchal cord, decreased fetal heart rate, acidosis, breech presentation, prematurity
- Postdelivery: asphyxia, neonatal seizures, apnea, jaundice, postnatal infections, Apgar score below 5 at 5 minutes

Cerebral palsy is a static, nonprogressive syndrome. Degenerative diseases must be excluded in those who appear to be losing function. Cerebral palsy is divided into four types, which are described below, depending on the site of damage.

SPASTIC QUADRIPLEGIA

All four limbs are affected.

Etiology

- Intrauterine disease
- Cerebral malformations
- Hypoxic-ischemic damage in a full term infant

Early Manifestations

- Seizures in the first 24 to 48 hours of life, especially with hypoxic-ischemic encephalopathy
- Poor socialization
- Poor head control
- May be hypotonic in infancy
- Increased deep tendon reflexes, clonus, Babinski
- Cortical thumbs

Later Manifestations

- Delayed milestones
- Microcephaly
- Seizures often seen
- Mental retardation
- Fisting (cortical thumbs)
- Diffuse increased tone
- Increased deep tendon reflexes, clonus, Babinski
- Poor swallowing (may require gastrostomy)
- May never walk or sit alone

Pathology

Diffuse neuronal necrosis

Differential Diagnosis

If prenatal or perinatal distress is not present, exclude congenital malformations, hydrocephalus, metabolic abnormality, and, if the child's condition is deteriorating, leukodystrophy.

HEMIPARETIC CEREBRAL PALSY

Weakness is seen on one side of the body.

Etiology

The etiology is usually vascular (intrauterine): either hemorrhage or cerebrovascular accident or cerebral malformations.

Early Manifestations

- Fisting on the affected side
- Early handedness: lateralization before 1 year of age
- Does not bear weight on the affected side
- Up on toes on the affected side
- Delayed sitting (falls over as affected leg hyperextends)
- May not be recognized until 5 to 6 months of age or later
- May have homonymous hemianopsia

Later Manifestations

- Delayed milestones
- Limited facial weakness

- Hemiparesis
- May have hemiatrophy (if parietal involvement is present)—due to sensory loss ("trophic factor")
- Usually walks independently by 3 years of age
- Sensory loss: minimal
- Occurrence of seizures: variable; these usually develop in the first 2 years of life
- Intelligence may or may not be affected
- Requires bracing and surgery for tight heel cords
- Value of Botox still being debated
- Physical therapy

Pathology

- Arterial occlusion leading to infarction (greater risk with maternal cocaine use)
- Infarction
  - More often full-term infants
  - Watershed distribution (often associated with resuscitation)
  - Multiarterial infarction (congenital heart disease, polycythemia, disseminated intravascular coagulation)
  - Single artery infarction; trauma to neck—more than likely unknown
- Porencephalic cyst
- Cerebral malformation (heterotopias)
- Ventricle enlarged on side of lesion
- Hemispheric atrophy

Differential Diagnosis

The presence of a congenital brain tumor, which is also associated with early handedness, must be excluded. More often with tumors, the child will be ambidextrous for several months before he or she acquires handedness, as opposed to a static encephalopathy where the child has always had a hand preference. Increased head circumference suggests a mass lesion.

SPASTIC DIPLEGIA

All four limbs are affected, and the legs are much more involved than the arms.

Etiology

- Hypoxic-ischemia and hypotension in premature infants
- Associated with prematurity

Early Manifestations

- Alert and social
- Hands open, no fisting, arms relatively spared
- Increased tone in legs, especially hip adductors, hamstrings, and gastrocnemius
- Increased deep tendon reflexes in the lower extremities, clonus, Babinski
- Delay in sitting: extends legs when pulled to sit
- "Scissors" when put in standing position (contractions of the adductor muscles) and up on toes
- Strabismus often seen

Later Manifestations

- Delayed motor milestones
- Usually normal intelligence
- Usually no seizures
- Clumsy hands, but function adequately
- May walk independently but usually requires bracing, antispasticity medications, rhizotomy, or Botox to maximize benefits from physical therapy

Pathology

Periventricular leukomalacia and/or intraventricular hemorrhage

Differential Diagnosis

If the arms are normal and the history is unclear (particularly if the child is not premature), the patient must be evaluated as if he or she has paraplegia. Exclude the presence of a spinal cord lesion (tumor, transection), a parasagittal lesion, or hydrocephalus (placing pressure on periventricular leg fibers).

CHOREOATHETOTIC CEREBRAL PALSY

Etiology

- Kernicterus
- Sudden hypoxic-ischemic episode as in uterine rupture (placenta abruptio)

Early Manifestations

- No choreoathetosis in the first 2 years of life
- Often hypotonic

- Delayed motor milestones
- Normal socialization
- Obligate tonic neck
- Splaying of fingers when reaching
- Neurosensory deafness (if the etiology is kernicterus)

Later Manifestations

- Choreoathetosis
- Difficulty with speech
- Often drools
- Intelligence can be normal
- May or may not walk independently
- May require communication devices

Pathology

Status marmoratus (marbleization of basal ganglia secondary to faulty myelination)

Differential Diagnosis

Because choreoathetosis presents late (between the ages of 2 to 3 years), degenerative disease, aminoacidopathies, organic acidurias, Hallervorden-Spatz, and dopamine-sensitive choreoathetosis must be excluded.

Suggested Reading

Bushan V, Paneth N, Kiely J. Impact of improved survival of very low birth weight infants on recent secular events in the prevalence of cerebral palsy. *Pediatrics* 1993;91:1094–1100.

Edgar TS. Clinical utility of botulinum toxin in the treatment of cerebral palsy: comprehensive review. *J Child Neurol* 2001;16:37–46.

Freeman JM, Nelson KB. Intrapartum asphyxia and cerebral palsy. *Pediatrics* 1988;82:240–249.

Hill A. Current concepts of hypoxic-ischemic cerebral injury in the term newborn. *Pediatr Neurol* 1991;7:317–325.

Kuban KC, Leviton A. Cerebral palsy [review]. *N Engl J Med* 1994;330: 188–195.

Nelson KB, Ellenberg JH. Antecedents of CP: univariate analysis of risks. *Am J Dis Child* 1985;139:1031–1038.

Nelson KB, Ellenberg JH. Children who "outgrew" cerebral palsy. *Pediatrics* 1982;69:529–536.

Nelson KB, Grether JK. Causes of cerebral palsy. *Curr Opin Pediatr* 1999;11:487–491.

Paternak JF, Gorey MT. The syndrome of acute near-total intrauterine asphyxia in the term infant. *Pediatr Neurol* 1998;18:391–398.

Volpe JJ. *Neurology of the newborn,* 3rd ed. Philadelphia: WB Saunders, 1995.

Wilson-Costello D, Borawski E, Friedman H, et al. Perinatal correlates of cerebral palsy and other neurologic impairment among very-low-birth-weight children. *Pediatrics* 1998;102:315–322.

Chapter 12

Hemiparesis and Stroke

Case

A 10-year-old girl presents with left-sided weakness involving the face and the arm greater than the leg. After the onset of the weakness, she complained of a right-sided headache. Family history is significant for her mother having similar episodes of headache and hemiparesis. Magnetic resonance imaging (MRI) and magnetic resonance angiography (MRA) are normal.

Diagnosis

Familial hemiplegic migraine
The hemiplagia resolved after 48 hours.

DEFINITION OF HEMIPARESIS

Weakness is seen in one side of body, including the face, arm, and leg.

General Characteristics

- Weakness involves both the pyramidal and extrapyramidal motor systems.
- Arm contralateral to the lesion tends to be flexed at the elbow and wrist.
- Arm swing is decreased when walking. The involved leg is circumducted with foot drop.
- A pronator sign is seen with the arms extended (affected arm will turn from supination to pronation and drift downward).

- Depending on degree of extrapyramidal involvement, dystonia may be present.
- Tone is increased on affected side with signs of spasticity (increased stretch reflexes with sudden give).
- Reflexes are increased with a Babinski sign on the affected side.
- Gait is characterized by decreased arm swing, flexion of arm at elbow, and foot drop

In Infants and Very Young Children

- Affected hand tends to be fisted.
- Elbow on the affected side tends to be flexed.
- When put in an upright position, child stands flatfooted on normal side and up on the toe of the affected side.
- Child does not bear weight well on his or her affected hand or foot.
- Moro reflex is asymmetric.
- Facial sparing suggests a prenatal onset.

HISTORY

Tempo and Progression

Sudden Onset: Vascular

- Emboli
- Central nervous system (CNS) bleed: rare
- Cortical vein thrombosis
- Occlusive arterial disease
- Hemiplegic migraine
- Epileptic postictal state (Todd paralysis)
  - Follows partial seizure
  - Neuronal exhaustion phenomenon
  - Typically clears after 24 to 48 hours
  - May last up to 1 week

Subacute

- Development over days to weeks: thrombosis (hours to days)
- Brain tumor
- Abscess

- Arteriovenous malformation
- Subdural hematoma

Chronic

- Static encephalopathy
- Low grade tumor
- CNS malformation

Other Historical Points

- Did hemiparesis develop *after* headache (consider CNS bleed or cerebrovascular accident) versus *preceding* the headache (consider hemiplegic migraine)?
- Did the patient have seizures (cortical location as opposed to brainstem or spinal cord)?
- Does the patient have a history of congenital heart disease, especially cyanotic (child under the age of 2 years)?
- Does the history indicate that the patient has been taking illicit drugs, especially cocaine, or birth control pills (increased risk of stroke)?

Physical Examination

- Detailed general examination, especially cardiac function, cardiac rhythm, blood pressure, and bruits.
- Assess for oral trauma.

Localization

Cortical Hemiparesis

- Face, arm, and leg are involved on the same side. If face and arm involvement is greater than that of the leg, the middle cerebral artery is implicated. If leg involvement is greater than that of the face and arm, then the anterior cerebral artery is implicated.
- Visual field abnormalities are seen in parietal involvement.
- Eyes tend to "look at lesion."
- Cortical sensory loss implies a parietal or subcortical location.
- Aphasia is seen with a left hemisphere lesion, except in 8% to 15% of left-handed individuals who may be right hemisphere dominant. Decreased speech output with normal comprehension is suggestive of a nonfluent aphasia that is localized to the

posterior frontal region (Broca aphasia). Fluent aphasia, or normal verbalization with poor comprehension, suggests posterior temporal localization (Wernicke aphasia).

- Despite localization, fluent aphasias are rare.
- Young children typically become mute regardless of the site of lesion, but they recover language if the insult occurs at younger than 5 to 7 years of age and, at times, up to younger than 12 years of age.

Subcortical

- Subcortical location (internal capsule, basal ganglia [globus pallidus, putamen] thalamus)
- Face, arm, and leg equally involved
- May be pure motor or pure sensory deficit.
- Lacunar infarcts: favorable prognosis in children.

Brainstem

- No aphasia
- Eyes "look at hemiparesis" and away from the lesion
- No visual field abnormalities
- Crossed signs at the level of the lesion: ipsilateral cranial nerves, contralateral long tracts
- Cerebellar signs (ipsilateral to lesion): finger to nose ataxia, difficulty with alternating hand movements

CAUSES OF STROKE IN CHILDREN

Stroke Secondary to Primary Vascular Disease

Acute Infantile Hemiplegia

- Infarction in middle cerebral artery (MCA), posterior cerebral artery (PCA), or anterior cerebral artery (ACA) distribution
- Sudden onset hemiparesis
  - Prolonged seizures, fever, coma in 60%
  - Acute hemiparesis without seizures or coma in 25%
  - Acute hemiparesis after brief seizure in 15%

Moyamoya Disease

- Basilar arterial occlusive disease
- Associated with multiple strokes and progressive dementia.

- Female predominance
- **Etiology**
  - Seen after cranial irradiation, especially to midline. Particular risk for children younger than 5 years of age with neurofibromatosis type 1 who are irradiated for optic pathway tumors
  - Down syndrome
  - Sickle cell disease
  - Idiopathic

Evaluation

- Computed tomography (CT), MRI (multiple strokes)
- Angiography—occlusion of supraclinoid portion of the internal carotid artery (ICA), MCA, ACA and posterior communicating artery (PCA); telangiectasia in basal ganglia

Treatment

Encephaloduroarteriosynangiosis

Alternating Hemiplegia Of Childhood

- Onset at less than 18 months of age
- Repeated episodes of hemiplegia or hemiparesis lasting minutes to days
- Associated with dystonic attacks
- Paroxysmal nystagmus or abnormal eye movements
- Autonomic disturbance
- Attacks often bilateral
- Going to sleep associated with disappearance of symptoms
- Association with mental retardation and regression
- Electroencephalogram, MRI, and cerebral arteriograms: normal

Fibromuscular Dysplasia

- Nonatheromatous angiopathy
- Rare in children
- "Beading" seen on angiography

Hemiplegic Migraine

- Transient focal neurologic deficits lasting hours to days
- Autosomal dominant (chromosome 19) in some families

Stroke Secondary to Cyanotic Congenital Heart Disease

- Venous sinus thrombosis
- Tetralogy of Fallot and transposition of the great vessels—most common
- Increases with dehydration and polycythemia
- Usually seen before 2 years of age; presents with acute hemiparesis, seizures, coma, and increased intracranial pressure (ICP).
- Hemiparesis: becomes bilateral
- Mortality and/or morbidity high in infancy

Evaluation

On MRI, a hemorrhagic infarction is seen adjacent to venous thrombosis.

Treatment

- Hydration
- Control the increased ICP with steroids
- Antibiotics

Stroke Secondary to Embolic Arterial Occlusion

- Acute hemiparesis, seizures, headache, and loss of consciousness
- Abrupt onset

Etiologies

- Rheumatic heart disease
  - Valvular vegetation—subacute bacterial endocarditis
  - Abscess secondary to subacute bacterial endocarditis and valvular vegetations—unusual in children younger than the age of 2 years
- Prosthetic valves
- Cardiac arrhythmias, especially atrial fibrillation
- Cyanotic heart disease—right to left shunt (emboli can bypass lungs and enter the brain directly)
- Cardiac surgery or catheterization
- Fat emboli
- Paradoxical embolus via patient foramen ovale
- Cardiac myxoma
- Cardiac rhabdomyoma (tuberous sclerosis)

Stroke Secondary to Dissection of Carotid or Vertebral Arteries

Etiologies

- Intraoral trauma
- Neck injuries
- Spontaneous

Symptoms

Recurrent transient ischemic attacks or strokes are seen.

Treatment

- Acute: low molecular weight heparin or unfractionated heparin
- Chronic: Coumadin for 3 to 6 months

Stroke Secondary to Hematologic Disorders

Antiphospholipid Antibodies

These (lupus anticoagulant and anticardiolipid antibody) predispose the patient to arterial or venous thrombosis. They are found in 50% of children with systemic lupus erythematosus.

- Primary antiphospholipid syndrome: recurrent thrombosis and antiphospholipid antibodies
- Hypercoagulable states
  - Antithrombin III, protein C, protein S (autosomal recessive), factor V Leiden
  - Prone to venous and arterial thrombosis
  - Seen with polycythemia vera, leukemia, and dehydration
  - Suspect inherited hypercoagulable state if recurrent venous thrombosis

Sickle Cell Anemia

- Cerebrovascular disease: develops in 25%
- Thrombotic stroke
- Hemorrhage: less common
- Narrowing or obliteration of the large and medium vessels due to intimal proliferation and sickling
- Occurs at times of crisis or due to progressive vasculopathy
- Focal or generalized seizures
- May develop Moyamoya disease

- **Treatment**
    - Chronic transfusions with proven vascular disease
    - Keep hemoglobin S less than 20% to 30% of normal hemoglobin

Stroke Secondary to Toxins

- Cocaine, lysergic acid diethylamide (LSD), and amphetamines may cause hypertension, vasospasm, and stroke.
- Birth control pills may increase the risk of stroke.
- L-Asparaginase may be associated with an increased risk of stroke.
    - Hemorrhagic or thrombotic stroke
    - Decreased fibrinogen leading to hemorrhage
    - Decreased antithrombin III, protein C, and plasminogen leading to thrombotic stroke

Stroke Secondary to Metabolic Disorders

- Lactic acidemia, organic acidemia, hyperammonemia
- Basal ganglia infarction: Leigh disease, methylmalonic acidemia, glutaric aciduria type II, sulfite oxidase deficiency
- MELAS syndrome: stroke syndromes in nonvascular distribution, elevation of lactic acid, ragged red fibers on muscle biopsy
- Homocystinuria
    - Error in methionine metabolism
    - Thrombotic syndrome
    - Increased platelet aggregation

Stroke Secondary to Oral Trauma

This is seen with injury to the tonsillar fossa or carotid artery in the neck (lollipop in mouth). The tonsillar fossa is anterior to the carotid sheath.

Stroke Secondary to Infectious Causes

- Bacterial meningitis with retrograde venous infarction
- Bacterial meningitis with arterial thrombosis
- Internal carotid artery thrombosis secondary to pharyngitis, retropharyngeal abscess, or cervical adenitis
- Cat scratch fever (vasculitis)
- Viral encephalitis (herpes simplex, Coxsackie virus 9, ophthalmic herpes zoster)
- Mycoplasma (vasculitis)

Stroke Secondary to Central Nervous System Hemorrhage

Vascular Malformations

Arteriovenous Malformations

- Arteries drain into venous channels directly.
- Parietal location is found in 30%.
- Patient may present with hemorrhage (subarachnoid, intraparenchymal, or both).
  - May be sudden or progressive
  - Headache and neck stiffness with *subarachnoid hemorrhage*
  - Focal signs with increased ICP if *intraparenchymal*
- Seizures are first symptom in one-third of patients.
  - Partial or secondarily generalized
  - Hemorrhage before diagnosis in 20% to 70%
- Headaches are seen in 70% of cases.
- **Evaluation**
  - CT, MRI, MRA
  - Angiography
- **Prognosis**
  - Mortality with first bleed in 5% to 25%
  - Rebleeding in 25% to 50% and increase in mortality to 40%.
  - Risk of rupture: 3% to 4% per year
  - Lesions less than 3 cm: increased risk of rupture
- **Treatment**
  - Supportive
  - Control ICP
  - Embolization
  - Excision
  - Gamma radiation

Venous Angiomas

- These are the most common asymptomatic vascular malformation.
- Multiple venous channels drain into a single vein.
- They do not require surgery.

Cavernous Angiomas

- Large venous channels forming a meshwork
- Often multiple ones in brain and other organs
- Frontal and parietal

- Positive family history (FH)
- Seizures, headaches, hemorrhage
- Risk of rupture: 0.25% to 0.7% per year
- No surgery unless recurrent bleed or progressive symptoms

Vein of Galen Malformation

- This is the most common arteriovenous malformation in neonates.
- A direct connection is found between the carotid or vertebral arteries and the vein of Galen.
- High output congestive heart failure may develop due to shunting.
  - Wide pulse pressure
  - Tachycardia
  - Hepatomegaly
  - Respiratory distress
- Cranial bruit is present.
- Cerebral ischemia may result.
- Some develop hydrocephalus secondary to aqueductal compression.
- **Treatment**
  - Embolism of malformation—sequential procedures
  - Treat heart failure

Aneurysms

- Rare in children
- Seventy-five percent: congenital; most in the anterior circulation
- Ten percent: infectious; congenital heart disease with subacute bacterial endocarditis
- Onset: sudden, severe headache (at time of rupture)
- Focal deficits, alteration in consciousness
- Meningismus
- Giant aneurysms (one-third of pediatric aneurysms)
- Associated conditions
  - Polycystic kidneys
  - Ehlers-Danlos
  - Marfan syndrome
  - Tuberous sclerosis
  - Coarctation of the aorta
  - Agenesis corpus callosum

Evaluation

- CT of the head
- Lumbar puncture
- MRI and MRA
- Angiography

Treatment

- Stabilize
- Surgery

Stroke Secondary to Venous Thrombosis

Etiologies

- Dehydration, especially hypernatremic
- Sickle cell disease
- Hypercoagulable states—deficiencies in protein C, protein S, antithrombin III; factor V Leiden deficiency; may also be due to L-asparaginase
- Cyanotic congenital heart disease
  - Polycythemia leading to increased viscosity
  - Decreased oxygen (O_2) transport
- Homocystinuria
- Malignancy
  - Neuroblastoma
  - Increased white blood cells in leukemia
- Infection
  - Meningitis
  - Mastoiditis leading to lateral sinus thrombosis
  - Periorbital, paranasal, or frontal sinus infection leading to cavernous sinus thrombosis

Clinical Presentation

- Generalized thrombosis: encephalopathy leading to confusion, headache, seizures, lethargy, and increased ICP
- Cavernous sinus thrombosis—involves cranial nerves II, IV, V (ophthalmic), and VI
- Sagittal sinus thrombosis
  - Seizures

- Bilateral hemiparesis
- Coma

■ Lateral sinus thrombosis
- Visual field loss
- Headache
- Pseudotumor cerebri

Evaluation

Conduct MRI, MRA, and magnetic resonance venography (MRV).

Treatment

- Supportive
- Steroids
- Anticoagulation: controversial

EVALUATION OF A CHILD WITH ACUTE HEMIPLEGIA

Laboratory

- MRI
- MRA
- Electroencephalogram
- Lumbar puncture after CT or MRI has ruled out focal mass lesion; cells; cytology; protein; and polymerase chain reaction (PCR) for herpes
- Urine for amino acids (homocystinuria)
- Cardiac echocardiogram, transesophageal echocardiogram (TEE)
- Holter tape
- Complete blood count, platelets (if anemic, do a sickle cell preparation)
- Antinuclear antibody
- Antithrombin III level, protein C, protein S, Factor V Leiden, and urine toxicology

Treatment

- Dependent on etiology
- Residual hemiparesis—requires physical and occupational therapy and speech therapy where indicated

Suggested Reading

Aicardi J. Alternating hemiplegia of childhood. *Int Pediatr* 1987;2:115–119.

Aicardi J, Goutières F. Les thromboses veineuses intracraniennes, complication des déshydratations aiguës du nourrisson. *Arch Franc Pediatr* 1973;30:809–830.

Brey RL, Hart RG, Sherman DG, et al. Antiphospholipid antibodies and cerebral ischemia in young people. *Neurology* 1990;40:1190–1196.

DeVeber G, Andrew M, Adams C, et al. Cerebral sinovenous thrombosis in children. *N Engl J Med* 2001;345:417–423.

Freedom RM. Cerebral vascular disorders of cardiovascular origin in infants and children. In: Edwards BS, Hoffman HJ, eds. *Cerebral vascular disease in children and adolescents.* Baltimore: Williams & Wilkins, 1989:423–428.

Furlan AJ, Breuer AC. Central nervous system complications of open heart surgery. *Stroke* 1984;15:912–919.

Gerosa M, Licata C, Fiore DL, et al. Intracranial aneurysms in childhood and adolescence. *Child Brain* 1980;6:295–302.

Golden GS. Cerebrovascular diseases. In: Swaiman KF, ed. *Pediatric neurology: principles and practice,* 2nd ed. St. Louis: Mosby-Year Book, 1994: 787–803.

Hauser RA, Lacey M, Knight MR. Hypertensive encephalopathy: magnetic resonance imaging demonstration of reversible cortical and white matter lesions. *Arch Neurol* 1988;45:1078–1083.

Meyer FB, Sundt TM, Fode FC, et al. Cerebral aneurysms in childhood and adolescence. *J Neurosurg* 1989;70:420–425.

Packer RJ, Rorke LB, Lange BJ, et al. Cerebrovascular accidents in children with cancer. *Pediatrics* 1985;76:194–201.

Pavlakis SG, Kingsley PB, Bialer MG. Stroke in children: genetic and metabolic issues. *J Child Neurol* 2000;15:308–315.

Pearl PL. Childhood stroke following intraoral trauma. *J Pediatr* 1987; 110:574–575.

Phornphutkul CL, Rosenthal A, Nadas AS. Cerebrovascular accidents in infants and children with cyanotic congenital heart disease. *Am J Cardiol* 1973;32:329–334.

Riela AR, Roach SR. Etiology of stroke in childhood. *J Child Neurol* 1993;8:201–220.

Roach ES, Riela AR. *Pediatric cerebrovascular disorders,* 2nd ed. New York: Futura, 1995.

Sarnaik SA, Lusher JM. Neurological complications of sickle cell anemia. *Am J Hematol Oncol* 1982;4:386–394.

Seligsohn U, Berger A, Abend M, et al. Homozygous protein C deficiency manifested by massive venous thrombosis in the newborn. *N Engl J Med* 1984;310:559–562.

Volpe JJ. *Neurology of the newborn,* 3rd ed. Philadelphia: WB Saunders, 1995.

Young RS, Coulter DL, Allen RJ. Capsular stroke as a cause of hemiplegia in infancy. *Neurology* 1983;33:1044–1046.

Chapter 13

Developmental Disabilities

Case

A 7-year-old boy is brought to the office with complaints of doing poorly in school. The child does not read at grade level, has difficulty with fine motor coordination, and has history of delay in developmental milestones. He did not walk until 18 months of age. He did not speak until 3 years of age. The mother has a GED diploma, and the father completed high school. The Weschler Infant Scale for Children reveals an intelligence quotient of 75.

Diagnosis

Educable to borderline intelligence

Developmental disabilities are loosely defined as either a failure or a lack of ability to acquire age-specific cognitive, motor, language, and social skills at the expected maturational age. Approximately 5% to 10% of preschool age children in the United States are considered developmentally disabled.

ETIOLOGIES

Intrauterine

- Toxins: alcohol, illicit drugs
- Infectious: toxoplasmosis, cytomegalovirus, herpes, rubella, human immunodeficiency virus

- Genetic: fragile X, trisomy 21
- Malformations: lissencephaly, migration disorders
- Poor maternal–fetal interaction (i.e., intrauterine growth retardation)

Perinatal

- Hypoxic ischemic encephalopathy
- Infection: herpes, bacterial meningitis
- Trauma
- Hyperbilirubinemia
- Hypoglycemia

Postnatal

- Inborn errors of metabolism
- Toxins
- Infection
- Trauma

Idiopathic

This is the most common etiology.

MEASURES OF INTELLIGENCE

Most of the standard tests have a mean of 100 with a standard deviation (SD) of 15 and a standard error of the mean of 5. Two SDs below the mean defines mental retardation.

Common developmental scales include the following:

- Bailey Scale of Infant Development: measures development in infants from the age of 1 month to 4 years
- Wechsler Intelligence Scale for Children: measures intelligence from 6 to 12 years of age
- Wechsler Intelligence Scale: measures 16 years of age and up
- Stanford-Binet Scale: evaluates those from 2.5 to 23 years of age
- Leiter International Scale (nonverbal): assesses children from the age of 2 to 18 years
- Peabody Picture Vocabulary Test: evaluates language in children from 2 to 6 years of age
- Wide range achievement tests: used from the ages of 5 years to adult

- Woodcock Johnson cycle educational battery: tests basic academic skills

DYSLEXIA

This is defined as an inability to read at age level despite normal intelligence, motivation, and available schooling. The prevalence varies from 5% to 20% of school-aged children.

Etiology

- Familial
- Trauma
- Drugs
- Specific neurologic syndromes (i.e., Williams syndrome)

Clues

- Difficulty with single word decoding
- Failure to identify form constancy of letters (i.e., m, n, u, v, w, b, p, and q)
- Phonologic difficulty (i.e., sounding out words)
- Poor spelling
- Comprehension that is out of proportion to decoding skills
- Poor word retrieval skills
- Slow reading
- Associated attention deficit disorder

DEVELOPMENTAL LANGUAGE DISORDERS

This is defined as verbal intelligence that is delayed or that often does not develop. Several types are seen as follows:

- Phonologic: speech problems are seen with motor deficits. Multiple sequencing errors are observed.
- Lexical and syntactic: speech is sparse. Paraphasias are common, and syntax is confused.
- Phonologic–syntactic: sounds and syntax are both poor in this syndrome. Speech tends to be telegraphic.
- Verbal auditory abnormalities: difficulty with both expression and reception is seen with this syndrome. Spoken language is noncommunicative.

- Semantic pragmatic: speech is fluid and syntax is correct in this situation, but comprehension and verbal reasoning are impaired.

MENTAL RETARDATION

This is defined by the World Health Organization as "incomplete or insufficient development of mental capacities." It is loosely defined as nonprogressive limitations of intellect, which are two SDs below most tests of intellectual function, with concurrent deficits in adaptive functioning.

Epidemiology

- Six to 20 per 1,000 population
- Two percent to 3% of school-aged children
  - Mild range of mental retardation: 85%
  - Moderate range of mental retardation: 7% to 10%
  - Severely retarded: 1% to 5%
- Incidence higher in males than in females
- Mild retardation: more prevalent in lower socioeconomic groups
- Moderate and severe retardation: equally distributed across all socioeconomic groups

Classification

- Mild: two SDs below the mean; at least 55, but no greater than 70
- Moderate: three SDs below the mean; at least 35, but no greater than 55
- Severe: four SDs below the mean; at least 20, but no greater than 35
- Profound: five SDs below the mean; no greater than 20

Etiology

- Genetic (examples)
  - Fragile X (CGG triplicate repeat)
    - Predominantly males
    - Intelligence quotient less than 70
    - May have autistic features
    - Long face, large ears
    - Macroorchidism

- Williams syndrome (17q microdeletion)
  - Infantile hypercalcemia
  - Retardation
  - Supravalvular aortic stenosis
  - Unusual facies, elfin
- Prader-Willi syndrome (paternal deletion, 15q11–13)
  - Retardation
  - Short stature
  - Obesity
  - Neonatal hypotonia
- Angelman syndrome (maternal deletion, 15q11–13)
  - Seizures
  - "Happy puppet"
  - Retardation
  - Autistic features
  - Acquired microcephaly
- Rett syndrome (Xq28, mutation in MeCP2 gene) (see Chapter 14)
  - Girls
  - Failure of head growth (acquired microcephaly)
  - Stereotypies—hand wringing, hand flapping
  - Hyperventilation
  - Apnea
  - Seizures
  - Retardation
- Trisomy 21: Down syndrome
  - Hypotonia
  - Single transverse palmar crease
  - Brachycephaly
  - Antimongoloid slant (eyes)
  - Retardation
  - Short stature
  - Brushfield spots (iris abnormalities)
  - Cardiac defect
  - Duodenal atresia
  - Lymphoproliferative disorders
  - High incidence of Alzheimer disease

- Hypoxic-ischemic syndromes
  - Prenatal
  - Perinatal
  - Postnatal

- Trauma
- Intrauterine and postnatal meningitis and encephalitis
- Malnutrition
- Toxin—lead

Defects of Development

Neurulation (3 to 4 Weeks' Gestation)

- Anencephaly
- Encephalocele
- Myelomeningocele

Prosencephalic Formation (2 to 3 Months' Gestation)

- Holoprosencephalics
  - Alobar
  - Semilobar
  - Lobar
- Agenesis of corpus callosum
- Septooptic dysplasia

Neuronal Proliferation (3 to 4 Months' Gestation)

- Microcephaly
- Macrocephaly (Soto syndrome)
- Neurocutaneous syndromes

Neuronal Migration Disorders (3 to 5 Months' Gestation)

- Schizencephaly
  - Open cleft
  - Closed cleft
- Lissencephaly: pachygyria
- Heterotopias

Organizational Defects of the Central Nervous System (5 Months' Gestation to 7 Years' Postnatal)

- Cortical dysgenesis
- Trisomy 21
- Fragile X

Myelination Defects (Birth to Decades Postnatal)

- Amino and organic acidopathies

- Rubella
- Periventricular leukomalacia

Idiopathic

Suggested Reading

Fletcher JM, Shaywitz SE, Shaywitz BA. Co-morbidity of learning and attention disorders: separate but equal. *Pediatr Clin North Am* 1999; 46:885–897.

Menkes JH, Sarnat HB, eds. *Child neurology,* 6th ed. Philadelphia: Lippincott Williams & Wilkins, 2000.

Rapin I. *Children with brain dysfunction.* New York: Raven Press, 1982. International Review Child Neurology Series.

Volpe JJ. *Neurology of the newborn,* 3rd ed. Philadelphia: WB Saunders, 1995.

Chapter 14

Progressive Degenerative Disease

Case

A 3-month-old infant is evaluated because of irritability, stiffness, fever, and hypersensitivity to stimuli. He has recently developed multifocal seizures. Over the next 4 months, he is found to have a peripheral neuropathy, with an elevation in spinal fluid protein. Magnetic resonance imaging shows diffuse cerebral atrophy with possible calcifications in the basal ganglia. Lyosomal testing reveals a deficiency of galactocerebrosidase.

Diagnosis

Krabbe disease

Dementia is defined as regression from a previous level of function. This is differentiated from a failure to acquire or the slow acquisition of developmental milestones. The latter implies a static condition, whereas the former suggests a progressive disorder. Most progressive abnormalities present before the age of 2 years; however, others do not have their onset until well into the first 5 years of life.

ONSET BEFORE AGE 2

Disorders of Metabolism

Disorders of Amino Acids

- Phenylketonuria

- Maple syrup urine disease (branched-chain amino acids)
- Urea cycle abnormalities
- Homocystinuria

Disorders of Carbohydrate Metabolism

- Glycogen storage disease
- Fructose intolerance
- Galactosemia

Disorders Associated with Acidosis

- Multiple cocarboxylase deficiency (biotinidase deficiency)
- Isovaleric acidemia
- Propionic acidemia
- Methylmalonic acidemia
- Renal tubular acidosis
- Mitochondrial disorders

Features Common to Disorders of Metabolism

- Usually present in the first few weeks of life
- Seizures
- Become symptomatic as food is introduced into the diet
- Can be in the family history
- Developmental delay
- Features that suggest diagnosis
  - Acidosis
  - Reducing substance in the urine
  - Unusual odor
  - Sparse brittle hair
  - Visceromegaly

Disorders of Lysosomal Enzymes (see Chapter 23)

Storage Disease Without Visceromegaly

- G_{M2} gangliosidoses (Tay-Sachs, hexosaminidase A)
- Krabbe disease (galactocerebroside β-galactosidase)
- Glycoprotein abnormalities
  - Mannosidosis (mannosidase)
  - Fucosidosis (α-L-fucosidase)
  - Sialidosis (neuraminidase)

- I-cell disease
- Metachromatic leukodystrophy (arylsulfatase A)

Storage Disease with Visceromegaly

- Niemann-Pick disease (sphingomyelinase)
- Gaucher disease (glucocerebrosidase)
- G_{M1} gangliosidosis (β-galactosidase)
- Peroxisomal disorders
  - Adrenoleukodystrophy
  - Zellweger syndrome

Macrocephaly

- Canavan disease (*N*-acetyl aspartic acid)
- Alexander disease—defect not identified

Features Common to Disorders of Lysosomes

- Normal development initially
- Loss of milestones
- Seizures
- Cognitive decline
- Motor abnormalities
- Can be a part of the family history
- Features that suggest diagnosis
  - Small or large head
  - Optic atrophy
  - Retinal changes
  - Nystagmus
  - Irritability
  - Imaging characteristics
  - Visceromegaly

Disorders of Mucopolysaccharides (see Chapter 23)

Failure to Degrade Glycosaminoglycans

- Clinical features
  - Short Stature
  - Cataracts
  - Corneal clouding
  - Visceromegaly

  - Radiographic abnormalities
- Diseases
  - Hurler, Hunter, Scheie syndromes (mucopolysaccharidosis)
  - Sanfillipo syndrome, types A through D (mucopolysaccharidosis type III)
  - Morquio syndrome, types A and B (mucopolysaccharidosis type IV)

Mitochondrial Disorders

- Disorders of oxidation with a normal lactate-to-pyruvate ratio
  - Carnitine
  - Carnitine palmityl transferase deficiency
  - Pyruvate dehydrogenase complex
  - Multiple cocarboxylase deficiency
- Disorders of respiratory chain enzymes
  - Complex I to IV
  - MELAS (Mitochondrial encephalomyopathy, lactic acidosis, and stroke-like episodes)
  - MERRF (Myoclonic epilepsy with ragged red fibers)
- Features that suggest diagnosis
  - Acidosis
  - Multiorgan involvement
  - Abnormalities of the lactate-to-pyruvate ratio
  - Seizures
  - Encephalopathy
  - Muscle disease

Neuronal Ceroid Lipofuscinosis (Infantile to Adult Forms)

- Abnormal electroretinogram (ERG)
- Optic atrophy
- Macular—gray to dull red
- Retinal pigmentary changes
- Seizures
- Blindness late in infancy
- Dementia

Hallervorden-Spatz Disease

- Chromosome 20p
- Magnetic resonance imaging changes in the basal ganglion and substantia nigra (tiger eyes)

- Increased accumulation of iron in the basal ganglia
- Mutation in the gene for pantothenate kinase in a regulatory gene in the coenzyme A pathway
- Clinical features
  - Dystonia
  - Muscular rigidity
  - Choreoathetosis
  - Dementia
  - Retinitis pigmentosa

Infantile Neuroaxonal Dystrophy

- Motor regression
- Spasticity
- Optic atrophy
- Abnormal movements

Pelizaeus-Merzbacher Disease

- X-linked
- Oscillation of the eyes
- May present as spasmus nutans
- Seizures
- Optic atrophy
- Choreoathetosis
- Small head

Peroxisomal Disorders: Neonatal Adrenoleukodystrophy, Zellweger Syndrome

- Clinical features
  - Cataracts
  - Retinopathy
  - Seizures
  - Cranial neuropathies
  - Multiorgan involvement
- Increased very long chain fatty acids
  - Increased pipecolic acid
  - Increased phytanic acid—Refsum disease
- Decreased plasmalogen level
- Course characterized by early death or severe disability

ONSET AFTER THE AGE OF 2 YEARS

Many genetic enzymatic and genetic abnormalities that present in infancy may also present in early childhood or adult life. They include the following:

- G_{M2} gangliosidosis
- Gaucher disease
- Late onset Krabbe
- Niemann-Pick, type C
- Metachromatic leukodystrophy
- Adrenoleukodystrophy
- Neuronal ceroid lipofuscinosis
- Mitochondrial disorders

Disorders of Peroxisomes

- Adrenoleukodystrophy
  - Genetics
    - X-linked recessive: Xq28
    - Encodes peroxisomal membrane protein
  - Affects very long chain fatty acids, which accumulate in the plasma, brain, and testes
- Clinical features
  - Adrenal failure
  - Ataxia
  - Spasticity
  - Dementia
  - Bronze skin
  - Loss of vision
- Magnetic resonance imaging
  - Increased T2-weighted signals in the parietal occipital white matter
  - Atrophy of the cerebellum and pons
- Treatment
  - Treat the adrenal failure.
  - Diet should be rich in erucic or oleic acid.
  - Consider thalidomide, an antiinflammatory that is now in clinical trials.
  - Consider bone marrow transplantation.
  - Make a prenatal diagnosis with either amniocentesis or a chorionic villus biopsy.

Clues to Diagnosis

- Ocular abnormalities
  - Fundus: optic atrophy
    - Krabbe disease
    - Pelizaeus-Merzbacher disease
    - Metachromatic leukodystrophy (MLD)
  - Retinitis pigmentosa
    - Kearns-Sayre syndrome
    - Refsum disease
    - Cockayne syndrome
    - Hallervorden-Spatz disease
    - Neuronal ceroid lipofuscinosis
  - Cherry-red spot
    - Tay-Sachs
    - G_{M1} gangliosidosis
    - Niemann-Pick, types A and B
  - Macular abnormality—Batten disease
  - Sclera—Ataxia telangiectasia
  - Cataracts
    - Galactosemia
    - Myotonic dystrophy
    - Rubella
    - Down syndrome
  - Chorioretinitis
    - Cytomegalovirus
    - Rubella
  - Corneal clouding—Mucopolysaccharidosis
- Seizures
- Absent reflexes with Babinski responses
  - Krabbe disease
  - MLD
  - Adrenoleukodystrophy (ALD)
- Visceromegaly—storage disorder
- Acidosis—mitochondrial disease
- Dementia
- Head size
  - Increased head size
    - Canavan disease
    - Alexander disease
    - Most storage diseases

  - Decreased head size
    - Rett syndrome
    - Krabbe disease
- Hepatosplenomegaly
  - Niemann-Pick
  - Gaucher disease
  - Hurler syndrome
  - G_{M1} gangliosidosis
  - Glycogen storage disease

Evaluation

- Urine
  - Amino acids
  - Reducing substances—galactose
  - Dermatan sulfate and heparin sulfate for mucopolysaccharidosis
  - Sulfatides in MLD
- Serum
  - Amino acids
  - DNA testing
  - Galactose
  - Pyruvate and lactate levels
  - Lysosomal enzymes
  - Very long chain fatty acids
  - Copper, ceruloplasmin
    - Wilson disease
    - Menkes syndrome
- Muscle biopsy
  - Ragged red fibers
  - Dystrophies
  - Myopathies
  - Neuropathies
  - Inflammatory myopathy
- Bone marrow—look for foam cells, which are seen in Gaucher disease

DEGENERATIVE DISEASES NOT PRESENTING IN INFANCY

- Huntington disease
- Wilson disease

- Multiple sclerosis
- Juvenile Parkinson disease
- Subacute sclerosing panencephalitis

Suggested Reading

Aicardi J. The inherited leukodystrophies: a clinical overview. *J Inherit Metab Dis* 1993;16:733–743.

Allen RJ, McCusker JJ, Tourtellotte WW. Metachromatic leukodystrophy: clinical, histochemical, and cerebrospinal fluid abnormalities. *Pediatrics* 1962;30:629.

Baram TZ, Goldman AM, Percy AK. Krabbe disease: specific MRI and CT findings. *Neurology* 1986;36:111–115.

Brady RO, Argoff CE, Pentchev PG. The Niemann-Pick diseases group. In: Rosenberg RN, Prusinor SB, DiMauro S, et al., eds. *The molecular and genetic basis of neurological disease.* Boston: Butterworth-Heinemann, 1993.

Burton BK. Inborn errors of metabolism. The clinical diagnosis in early infancy. *Pediatrics* 1987;79:359–369.

Cox RP, Chuang DT. Maple syrup urine disease: clinical and molecular genetic considerations. In: Rosenberg RN, Prusinor SB, DiMauro S, et al., eds. *The molecular and genetic basis of neurological disease,* 2nd ed. Boston: Butterworth-Heinemann, 1997:1175–1193.

DiMaura S, Bonilla E, Zeviani M, et al. Mitochondrial myopathies. *J Inherit Metab Dis* 1987;10:113–128.

Glew RH, Basu A, Prence EM, Remaley AT. Lysosomal storage diseases [Review]. *Lab Invest* 1985;53:250–269.

Johnson WG. Genetic heterogeneity of hexosaminidase-deficiency diseases. *Res Publ Assoc Res Nerv Ment Dis* 1983;60:215–237.

Kelly RI. Peroxisomal disorders. In: Walker WA, Durie P, Hamilton R, et al., eds. *Pediatric gastrointestinal disease.* Toronto: BD Becker, 2000: 1185–1290.

Koch R, Friedman EG. Accuracy of newborn screening programs for phenylketonuria. *J Pediatr* 1981;98:267–269.

Kolodny EH. The GM2 gangliosidoses. In: Rosenberg RN, Prusinor SB, DiMauro S, et al., eds. *The molecular and genetic basis of neurological disease,* 2nd ed. Boston: Butterworth-Heinemann, 1997:473–490.

Kolodny EH, Moser HW. Sulfatide lipidosis: metachromatic leukodystrophy. In: Stanbury JB, Wyngaarden JB, Fredrickson DS, et al., eds. *The metabolic basis of inherited disease,* 5th ed. New York: McGraw-Hill, 1983.

Kolodny EH, Raghavan S, Krivit W. Late-onset Krabbe disease (globoid cell leukodystrophy): clinical and biochemical features of 15 cases. *Dev Neurosci* 1991;13:232–239.

McKusick VA, Neufeld EF, Kelly TE. The mucopolysaccharide storage diseases. In: Stanbury JB, Wyngaarden JB. Fredrickson DS, eds. *The metabolic basis of inherited disease,* 4th ed. New York: McGraw-Hill, 1978.

Meikle PJ, Hopwood JJ, Clague AE, Carey WF. Prevalence of lysosomal storage disorders. *JAMA* 1999;281:249–254.

Menkes JH, Sarnat HB, eds. *Child neurology,* 6th ed. Philadelphia: Lippincott Williams & Wilkins, 2000.

Milunsky A, et al. Prenatal genetic diagnosis. *N Engl J Med* 1970;283: 1498–1504.

Mole S, Gardener M. Molecular genetics of the neuronal ceroid lipofuscinoses. *Epilepsia* 1999;40:29–32.

Moser HW. Peroxisomal disorders. In: Rosenberg RN, Prusinor SB, DiMauro S, et al., eds. *The molecular and genetic basis of neurological disease,* 2nd ed. Boston: Butterworth-Heinemann, 1997:273–314.

Neufeld EF, Muenzer J. The mucopolysaccharidoses. In: Scriver CR, Beaudet AL, Sly WS, Valle D, eds. *The metabolic basis of inherited disease,* 6th ed. New York: McGraw-Hill, 1989.

Neufeld EF, Muenzer J. The mucopolysaccharidoses. In: Scriver CR, Beaudet AL, Sly WS, et al., eds. *The metabolic and molecular basis of inherited disease,* 7th ed. New York: McGraw-Hill, 1995:2465–2494.

O'Brien JS. The gangliosidoses. In: Stanbury JB, Wyngaarden JB. Fredrickson DS, eds. *The metabolic basis of inherited disease,* 3rd ed. New York: McGraw-Hill, 1983.

Powers JM, Moser HW. Peroxisomal disorders: genotype, phenotype, major neuropathologic lesions and pathogenesis. *Brain Pathol* 1998; 8:101–120.

Rahman S, Blok RB, Dahl HH, et al. Leigh syndrome: clinical features and biochemical and DNA abnormalities. *Ann Neurol* 1996;39:343–351.

Rosenberg RN, Prusiner SB, DiMauro S, Barchi RL, eds. *The molecular and genetic basis of neurological disease,* 2nd ed. Boston: Butterworth-Heinemann, 1997:23–28.

Stansbie D, Wallace SJ, Marsac C. Disorders of the pyruvate dehydrogenase complex. *J Inherit Metab Dis* 1986;9:105–119.

Taggart JM. Inborn errors of cellular organelles: an overview. *J Inherit Metab Dis* 1987;10:3–10.

Wallace DC. Diseases of the mitochondrial DNA. *Annu Rev Biochem* 1992; 61:1175–1212.

Chapter 15

Neurocutaneous Syndromes

Case

A 6-month-old boy presents with episodes of massive myoclonic jerks that appear in flurries. These have been occurring several times a day for the past 2 weeks. Along with the seizures, he seems to be becoming less alert and he is losing motor milestones. His birth and past medical history are unremarkable. The family history is unremarkable. His examination is normal, with the exception of a single hypopigmented spot on the abdomen, which was seen with a Wood's lamp. An electroencephalogram (EEG) reveals a hypsarrhythmic pattern. Computed tomography (CT) of the head reveals calcification in a periventricular location, with a large lesion at the foramen of Monro. An echocardiogram of the heart reveals a rhabdomyoma, and a renal ultrasound reveals renal cysts.

Diagnosis

Tuberous sclerosis

TUBEROUS SCLEROSIS

Genetics

- Autosomal dominant, variable expression; new mutations in 58% to 68% of cases
- Two genotypes for tuberous sclerosis complex (TSC
  - TSCI: deletion on chromosome 9
  - TSCI: deletion on chromosome 16

Incidence

The incidence is one in 10,000 to 30,000 births.

Affected Organs

Skin

- Adenoma sebaceum (angiofibromas of the skin): cheeks, nasolabial folds, chin (age of onset is 3 to 15 years)
- Ash-leaf spots: earliest sign; these are hypopigmented areas that fluorescence under ultraviolet light
- Shagreen patch (lumbosacral region)—rough skin
- Periungual fibromas: rare before puberty
- Fibrous plaques on the forehead or scalp
- Depigmented hair
- Dental enamel pitting (seen in 75% to 100% adults with tuberous sclerosis)

Brain

- Tubers: cortical
- Subependymal nodules: along the ventricular walls
- Subependymal giant cell astrocytoma (classically at foramen of Monro); these may grow but they only rarely become malignant; may cause obstructive hydrocephalus

Eyes

- Retinal phakomas (astrocytic benign tumors)
  - Mulberry appearance
  - May calcify
  - On or near the optic nerve head
- Less common: depigmented retinal areas, hyaline or cystic nodules, iris coloboma, cataracts

Heart

Rhabdomyoma is found in 40% to 50% of patients.

Kidney

- Angiomyolipomas—in 50% to 80% of patients
- Renal cysts
- Increased blood pressure

Lung

- Infiltration with multicystic changes (especially women)
- Exertional dyspnea or spontaneous pneumothorax

Vascular

- Hemangiomas
- Small vessel dysplasia
- Aneurysms in the intracranial vessels and aorta (rare)

Clinical

Seizures

- Infantile spasms: most common
- Tonic or atonic
- Complex partial

Mental Retardation

Mental retardation is seen in 80% of patients who have had seizures. All retarded patients have seizures.

- Autism
- Hyperactivity
- Normal intelligence in up to one-third

Evaluation

- CT of the head
  - Abnormal in 85%
  - Calcified subependymal nodules
  - Cortical or subcortical areas of decreased density
- Magnetic resonance imaging of the head
  - Cortical and subcortical tubers
  - T2-weighted hyperintensity
- EEG
  - Hypsarrhythmia in infantile spasms
  - Focal seizure discharges
  - Multifocal seizure discharges
- Echocardiogram: rhabdomyomas
- Renal ultrasound

- ◆ Renal cysts
- ◆ Angiomyolipomas

- Chest x-ray: pulmonary cysts
- Bone x-rays: cystic and sclerotic changes of the ribs, hands, and feet

Treatment

- Seizure control: anticonvulsants, corticotropin, and occasionally surgery of the symptomatic tuber
- Giant cell astrocytoma: if necessary, shunt with or without surgical removal. No radiation or chemotherapy is indicated.

STURGE-WEBER

Genetics

Genetic inheritance is sporadic.

Incidence

The incidence of this condition is 1 in 50,000.

Affected Organs

Skin

- Hemangioma involving the ophthalmic division of the fifth cranial nerve (port wine stain), usually above the palpebral fissure, affecting the upper eyelid, frontal region, or both,
- The buccal mucosa, tongue, palate, and pharynx possibly involved
- Unilateral in 70%
- Present at birth

Central Nervous System

Venous angioma is found in the pia mater (ipsilateral to the facial hemangioma).

- Occipital most common
- Temporal
- Parietal
- Underlying cortex: neuronal loss, gliosis, and calcification

Eyes

Choroidal angioma may be present and may cause glaucoma.

Clinical

- Seizures; 75% to 90% have onset in the first months of life; partial with or without secondary generalization
- Homonymous hemianopsia (contralateral to the facial angioma)
- Hemiplegia: seen in 30% to 50% (contralateral to the facial angioma)
- Mental retardation: 50% (75% of those with seizures)
- Intracranial hemorrhage: does not occur
- Glaucoma: seen in 30%

Evaluation

- Findings on CT and skull film are neutral.
- Calcification "tram track" is present in the parieto-occipital. The calcification may not appear for months or years after birth.
- Atrophy and enlarged choroid plexus are found on the side of the pial angioma.
- In addition, draining veins are abnormal.
- Magnetic resonance imaging (MRI) with gadolinium shows pial angioma, abnormal white matter, and thickened cortex.
- EEG shows reduced background amplitude with or without seizure discharges (affected side).
- Intraocular pressure should be monitored.

Treatment

- Seizure control should be attempted because hemiplegia is generally postconvulsive. Hemispherectomy should be done if anticonvulsants fail
- Laser treatment of port wine stain is indicated.
- Daily aspirin to prevent venous and capillary thrombosis has been recommended by some authors. No double-blind studies have been conducted.

LINEAR SEBACEOUS NEVUS SYNDROME

Affected Organs

Skin

- Slightly raised, yellow-orange, smooth linear plaque seen in the midline of the forehead, nose, or lip; later becomes darker and verrucous; may not be visible at birth

- Skin lesions: potentially malignant

Brain

- Hamartomatous tumors
- Porencephaly
- Arterial aneurysms
- Hemimeganencephaly

Eyes

- Dermoids or epidermoids of conjunctiva
- Colobomas of the iris, choroid, retina, or optic nerve
- Microphthalmia

Clinical

- Seizures
  - Partial
  - Infantile spasms
- Hemihypertrophy of the face, head, and limbs; may be present at birth or might develop over time
- Hemiplegia and/or hemianopia contralateral to the nevus (common)
- Mental retardation

Evaluation

- CT: may indicate hypertrophy in one hemisphere, a decreased size of the ipsilateral ventricle, and pachygyria with hypodense white matter
- EEG: may show paroxysmal activity and unilateral slowing. Hemihypsarrhythmia may occur.

NEUROFIBROMATOSIS TYPE 1

Genetics

Inheritance is autosomal dominant. One-third of cases represent new mutations.

Prevalence

The prevalence is 1 in 2,000 to 4,500 individuals.

Pathology

Dysplasia, with or without neoplasia, of the organs derived from the following:

- Embryonic ectoderm (skin, central nervous system, peripheral nervous system, eyes)
- Embryonic mesoderm (blood vessels, bone, cartilage)

Definitions of Neurofibromatosis

At least two of the following must be present

- At least five café-au-lait macules more than 5 mm diameter; if prepubertal, then at least six café-au-lait macules that are more than 15 mm diameter
- Two or more neurofibromas of any type or one plexiform neurofibroma
- Freckles in the axillary or inguinal regions
- Sphenoid wing dysplasia or congenital bowing of the long bone cortex, with or without pseudoarthrosis
- Bilateral optic nerve gliomas
- More than two Lisch nodules in the iris on slit-lamp examination
- A first-degree relative with neurofibromatosis

Affected Organs

Skin

- Café au lait
  - Oval
  - Smooth borders
  - Sharply demarcated
- Axillary freckling
- Inguinal freckling

Eyes

Lisch nodules appear in the iris with slit-lamp examination. They are seen in 30% of patients by 6 years of age; they appear in 100% of patients older than 12 years of age.

Peripheral Neurofibromas

- Increase with age
- Cutaneous: molluscum fibrosum

- Subcutaneous: discrete neurofibromas
- Both cutaneous and subcutaneous: plexiform neurofibromas
    - Disfiguring, gigantism
    - Massive size
    - Increased with age
    - Risk of malignant degeneration (malignant neurofibrosarcoma)

Central Tumors

- Optic nerve glioma
    - Most common brain tumor in the first decade of life
    - Bilateral optic gliomas: 100% have neurofibromatosis, type 1; may be asymptomatic
    - With good visual acuity and no increase in intracranial pressure: may be followed without treatment
- Brainstem glioma
- Astrocytoma
- Ependymoma

Spinal Cord

- Dural ectasia
- Extramedullary intradural tumors: neurofibromas, meningiomas
- Intramedullary tumors: astrocytomas, ependymomas (infrequent)
- Syringomyelia
- Hyperpigmented patches over the midline of the back: underlying neurofibroma of the spinal cord or nerve roots

Hydrocephalus

- Aqueductal stenosis
- Tectal tumors
- Other tumors obstructing the cerebrospinal fluid pathway

Bone

- Kyphoscoliosis
- Tibial (fibular) bowing
- Pseudoarthrosis
- Thinning of the long bone cortex
- Pathologic fractures

- Macrocephaly with head circumference greater than the 98th percentile
- Sphenoid wing dysplasia

Endocrine

- Precocious puberty
- Short stature
- Pheochromocytoma: 10% of patients with pheochromocytomas have neurofibromatosis, type 1

Pulmonary
Interstitial fibrosis is seen.

Vascular

- Arterial occlusive disease
  - Renal artery stenosis (increased blood pressure)
  - Moyamoya disease: basilar arterial occlusive disease (brain)
    - Highest risk: children younger than 5 years of age who are irradiated for optic pathway tumors
    - Multiple strokes
- Migraine

Other

- Mental retardation: 8%
- Learning disabilities: 40%
- Epilepsy: approximately 10%
- Cancer: in addition to central nervous system tumors, also develop leukemia, breast cancer, pheochromocytomas, and visceral tumors

Evaluation

- History and physical
  - Growth
  - Pubertal status
  - Scoliosis
  - Blood pressure
- Neurologic examination
- Visual acuity and visual fields
- Hearing (brainstem auditory-evoked response [BAER], audiogram)

- Educational evaluation
- MRI of the head and orbits
  - Unidentified bright objects ("UBOs"): increased T2-weighted signals in the basal ganglia, optic pathway, brainstem, and cerebellum; seen in 60% to 70% of patients
  - Decrease in number over time
  - Associated with learning disabilities

NEUROFIBROMATOSIS, TYPE 2

This condition is rare in children.

Genetics

- Autosomal dominant
- Chromosome 22

Prevalence

The prevalence of this condition is 1 in 30,000 to 50,000.

Affected Organs

Skin

Less than five café-au-lait spots are seen.

Brain

- Bilateral acoustic neuromas (90% of cases)
  - Late adolescence and adulthood
  - Bilateral deafness
- Meningiomas (multiple)
- Schwannomas in cranial nerves V to XII

Spinal Cord

- Schwannomas
- Ependymomas
- Meningiomas

Eyes

Cataracts are seen.

ATAXIA TELANGIECTASIA

Genetics

- Autosomal recessive
- Genetic abnormality on chromosome 11.q 22–23

Incidence

The incidence is 1 in 40,000 births.

Affected Systems

Skin

Telangiectasia is present.

- Onset from 2 to 10 years of age
- Bulbar conjunctiva seen first
- Upper half of the ears
- Flexor surfaces of the limbs
- Butterfly distribution on the face
- Increased by sun exposure

Brain

Degeneration of the Purkinje and granule cells in the cerebellum is seen.

Clinical Features

- Progressive truncal ataxia beginning in the first year of life
- Choreoathetosis
- Oculomotor apraxia in 90% of patients
- Dull or expressionless face
- Dysarthria
- Progressive dementia: one-third have mild mental retardation
- Recurrent sinopulmonary infections
- Growth failure
- Females: delayed or absent secondary sex characteristics
- Males: hypogonadism
- Liver dysfunction in 40% to 50%
- Metabolic glucose abnormalities in more than 50%

Evaluation

- Check serum and salivary immunoglobulin A (IgA)
- IgE absent or decreased in 80% to 90%
- IgM may be increased
- Increased α-fetoprotein
- Increased carcinoembryonic antigen
- T-cell deficiency in 60%
- Excessive chromosome breaks; translocations usually involve chromosomes 7 and 14
- Increased incidence of leukemia and lymphoma

Course

- Two-thirds die by the age of 20 years
  - Infection
  - Malignancy
  - Lymphoreticular malignancies
- Most patients wheelchair bound by 10 to 15 years of age
- Requires vigorous treatment of infections and pulmonary hygiene
- Radiation: possibly increases malignancies
- Limit radiologic studies

VON HIPPEL-LINDAU DISEASE

Genetics

- Autosomal dominant with high penetrance
- Gene mapped to distal short arm of chromosome 3 (3p25–26)

Incidence

This condition occurs in 1 in 39,000 live births.

Clinical

- Retinal hemangioblastomas
  - Children of at least 5 years of age
  - Intracranial tumor: 10%
  - May cause decreased vision from hemorrhage
- Cerebellar hemangioblastomas

  - Seen in 60% of patients
  - Polycythemia possibly associated
  - Usually develop at more than 15 years of age
- Hemangiomas in the brainstem, spinal cord, cerebral hemispheres: less frequent
- Renal lesions
  - Cysts
  - Adenomas
  - Hemangiomas
  - Malignant hypernephromas
  - Renal cell carcinomas: 28%
- Pancreatic cysts, hepatic cysts, splenic cysts
- Pheochromocytoma: 7%
- Adrenal adenoma: less common

Evaluation

- MRI of the brain to rule out cerebellar tumor
- Complete blood count to rule out polycythemia

Treatment

- Surgical removal of cerebellar hemangioblastoma
- Laser surgery for retinal hemangioblastoma

Patients and Others At Risk

- Yearly eye examinations
- Annual urinary screen for vanillylmandelic acid (VMA) and noradrenaline after 10 years of age
- Head MRI every 2 years when older than 15 years of age
- Abdominal CT when over 20 years of age

Suggested Reading

Abadir R, Hakami N. Ataxia-telangiectasia with cancer: an indication for reduced radiotherapy and chemotherapy doses. *Br J Radiol* 1983;56: 343–345.

Boder E. Ataxia-telangiectasia: an overview. In: Gatti RA, Swift M, eds. *Ataxia-telangiectasia: genetics, neuropathology and immunology of a degenerative disease of childhood.* New York: Alan R Liss, 1985:1–63.

Couch V, Lindor NM, Karnes PS, et al. von Hippel-Lindau disease. *Mayo Clin Proc* 2000;75:265–272.

DeBella K, Szudek J, Friedman JM. Use of the National Institutes of Health criteria for diagnosis of neurofibromatosis I in children. *Pediatrics* 2000;105:608–614.

Duffner PK, Cohen ME. Isolated optic nerve gliomas in children with and without neurofibromatosis. *Neurofibromatosis* 1988;1:201–211.

Duffner PK, Cohen ME, Seidel FG, et al. The significance of MRI abnormalities in children with neurofibromatosis. *Neurology* 1989;39:373–378.

Evans JC, Curtis J. The radiological appearances of tuberous sclerosis. *Br J Radiol* 2000;73:91–98.

Filling-Katz MR, Choyke PL, Oldfield E, et al. Central nervous system involvement in von Hippel-Lindau disease. *Neurology* 1991;41:41–46.

Friedrich CA. von Hippel-Lindau syndrome: a pleomorphic condition. *Cancer* 1999;86:1658–1662.

Levinsohn PM, Mikhael MA, Rothman SM. Cerebrovascular changes in neurofibromatosis. *Dev Med Child Neurol* 1978;20:789–793.

National Institutes of Health Consensus Development Conference. Neurofibromatosis conference statement. *Arch Neurol* 1988;45:575–578.

Packer RJ, Savino PJ, Bilaniuk LT, et al. Chiasmatic gliomas in childhood: reappraisal of natural history and effectiveness of cranial radiation. *Child Brain* 1983;10:393–403.

Prensky AL. Linear sebaceous nevus. In: Gomez MR, ed. *Neurocutaneous diseases: a practical approach.* London: Butterworth-Heineman, 1987: 335–344.

Roach ES, Riela AR, McLean WT, Stump DA. Aspirin therapy for Sturge-Weber syndrome. *Ann Neurol* 1985;18:387.

Roach ES, DiMario FJ, Kandt RS, et al. Tuberous Sclerosis Consensus Conference: recommendations for diagnostic evaluation. *J Child Neurol* 1999;14:401–407.

Sujansky E, Conradi S. Sturge-Weber syndrome: age of onset of seizures and glaucoma and the prognosis for affected children. *J Child Neurol* 1995;10:49–58.

Tallman B, Tan OT, Morelli JG, et al. Location of port-wine stains and the likelihood of ophthalmic and/or central nervous system complications. *Pediatrics* 1991;87:323–327.

Tomsik TA, Lukin RR, Chambers AA, et al. Neurofibromatosis and intracranial arterial occlusive disease. *Neuroradiology* 1976;11:229–234.

Werteleki W, Rouleau GA, Superneau DW, et al. Neurofibromatosis 2: clinical and DNA linkage studies of a large kindred. *N Engl J Med* 1988;319:278–283.

Chapter 16

Infectious Disease

Case

A 1-week-old infant is seen in the newborn nursery. He is lethargic and febrile, and he has a bulging fontanelle. He then develops seizures. Complete blood count reveals a high white count and thrombocytopenia, and the cerebrospinal fluid (CSF) is positive for *Listeria monocytogenes.*

Diagnosis

Neonatal meningitis

MENINGITIS, MENINGOENCEPHALITIS, AND ENCEPHALITIS

Meningitis by definition is the involvement of the meninges without the involvement of the parenchyma. Although meningoencephalitis implies the involvement of both the meninges and the cerebral parenchyma, encephalitis implies involvement of the brain parenchyma with sparing of the meninges. Abscess, on the other hand, is defined as a localized collection of pus; it has a very different pathophysiology from that of meningitis or encephalitis.

In bacterial meningitis, a minimal cellular response with no organism suggests the presence of overwhelming infection. In fungal meningitis, the CSF may have both polynuclear and mononuclear cells. Remember, although small numbers of mononuclear cells are part of the normal spinal fluid formula, the presence of even one polynuclear cell suggests a blood-borne process. Low sugar is always associated with active phagocytosis, and it suggests a bacterial infection until proven otherwise. In most bacterial infections of the nervous system, the sugar is below 20 regardless of the blood sugar level. The reduction of spinal fluid sugar more commonly profiles blood sugar so that a CSF sugar level of less than 40% of the blood sugar is usually suggestive of a central nervous system infection. Table 16.1 distinguishes among these.

Usual Bacterial Agents Seen in Childhood Meningitis

- Newborn
  - *Escherichia coli*
  - *L. monocytogenes*
  - Group B streptococcus
- Over 1 Month of Age
  - *Streptococcus pneumoniae*
  - *Neisseria meningitides*
  - *Haemophilus influenza:* less common with the advent of vaccine

The incidence of meningitis peaks at about 2 years of age. Less than 25% of the cases are found after 2 years of age.

Clinical Features

- Newborn
  - May be nonspecific (remember the "organs of the very young do not cry"). The only symptoms may be irritability, lethargy, failure to feed, and a high-pitched cry.
  - Specific signs: fever, seizures, and bulging fontanelle
  - Lumbar puncture: strongly recommended in children younger than 12 months of age with fever and seizure

TABLE 16.1 Cerebrospinal Fluid in Meningitis

	Bacteria	Viral	Fungal	Mycobacterium
Cells	++++	++	++	+++
Cell type	Polynuclear	Mononuclear	Mononuclear or polynuclear	Mononuclear
Sugar	↓↓ to ↓↓↓↓	Normal	↓↓	↓↓
Protein	↑↑	↑	↑↑	↑↑
Organism	Readily cultured	Difficult to recover	Variable	Recoverable

- Children over 2 years of age
  - Clinical signs: more specific
  - Include fever, stiff neck, and Brudzinski sign (flexion of the neck produce flexion of the knee and hip) with or without Kernig sign (pain in back on flexion of the thigh with extension of the knee)

Neurologic Complications of Meningitis

- Seizures: usually occur in the first 24 to 48 hours and resolve after 2 or 3 days. *For seizures that occur late in the course of the disease, a specific etiology for the seizure should be sought, such as an electrolyte imbalance, vasculitis, cerebritis, infarct, subdural empyema, or effusion (syndrome of inappropriate secretion of antidiuretic hormone).*
- Arterial vasculitis: develops with the most exudative meningitides (i.e., pneumococcus and staphylococcus). Tuberculous meningitis is also associated with a vasculopathy.
- Cortical vein thrombosis: occurs, as with arterial disease, with those meningitides that produce the most exuberant inflammatory reaction. Signs of cortical vein thrombosis are hemiparesis, seizures, long tract signs, and cognitive impairment.
- Cerebritis: seen in those meningitides that are not treated early or for which overwhelming infection that does not respond to antibiotics is present. Signs are as follows:
  - Cognitive defects
  - Seizures
  - Retardation
- Hydrocephalus: occurs as a complication of meningitis and results from adhesions at the base of the brain.
  - Communicating hydrocephalus: secondary to basal arachnoiditis
  - Noncommunicating hydrocephalus: secondary to obstruction of the cerebral spinal outflow tracks, usually at the level of the aqueduct
- Electrolyte imbalance
  - Seizures with hyponatremia (syndrome of inappropriate secretion of antidiuretic hormone)
  - Hemorrhage with hypernatremia
- Cranial neuropathies: usually a long-term consequence of meningitis. They are primarily seen in partially treated meningitis or in meningitis associated with delay in treatment. Signs are as follows:

  - Hearing loss: may be sudden or slowly progressive
  - Seventh nerve paresis
  - Optic neuropathy
- Subdural effusions: occur late. They usually require no treatment, and they are usually not associated with symptomatology.

Tuberculous Meningitis

- Look for extracranial source: pulmonary, renal, or miliary
- Subacute onset
  - Low grade fever
  - Headache
  - Lethargy
  - Behavioral changes

Fungal Meningitis

- This is uncommon, usually seen in immunologically compromised patients.
- Signs may mimic those of tuberculosis.
- CSF formula is similar to that of tuberculous meningitis: monocytic response, no bacterial growth, low sugar, and increased protein.

Viral or Aseptic Meningitis

- Acute onset, stiff neck, and fever
- Pain on movement of the eyes
- Sterile spinal fluid with normal sugar
- Seasonal: primarily seen in late summer, early fall
- Usually resolves without residual effects

ENCEPHALITIS

Viral encephalitis presents with systemic signs of infection, such as fever, tachycardia, and rash, in addition to signs and symptoms reflecting gray and white matter disease. These may include altered mental status, delirium, seizures, long tract signs, and, in more severe cases, brainstem involvement with respiratory compromise.

The course is variable. Children may recover completely, or they can be left with cognitive impairment and seizures. The diagnosis is based on CSF findings, polymerase chain reaction (PCR) for specific antigens, and acute and convalescent sera.

Over 100 viral agents are associated with encephalitis. Despite this daunting number, relatively few species of viruses are identified in children who present with an encephalopathic picture. The most significant DNA viruses are those belonging to the herpes family, whereas the most common RNA viruses belong to the picornaviruses.

Herpes simplex is the most common identifiable virus in childhood. As such, its clinical course is described. The others are listed but are not described as most do not have identifying features (Table 16.2).

Herpes Simplex

- Clinical features
  - Headache, vomiting, and lethargy
  - Systemic signs of infection variable
  - Hemiparesis
  - Aphasia
  - Seizures: focal or generalized
  - May progress to coma
- Diagnosis
  - PCR for herpes antigen in the CSF
  - Magnetic resonance imaging (MRI)
    - Increased T2 signal in temporal lobes, insula, and cingulate gyrus
    - Gadolinium-enhanced T1 signal in temporal lobe
  - Electroencephalogram
    - Focal or generalized slowing
    - Periodic epileptiform discharges that may be lateralizing

TABLE 16.2 Prominent Viruses of Medical Consequence

DNA Virus	RNA Virus
Herpes family	Picorna viruses
Herpes simplex	Polio
Cytomegalovirus	Echovirus
Varicella-zoster	Coxsackie
Epstein-Barr	Eastern and Western equine encephalitis
Adenovirus	St. Louis encephalitis
Hepatitis B	Rubella
	Mumps
	Rubeola
	Rabies

- Treatment: Give acyclovir for 10 to 14 days and monitor renal function.
- Course
  - Neurologic residual effects seen in up to 40% of cases, including the following:
    - Seizures
    - Motor deficits
    - Language and cognitive problems
    - Memory disturbances
    - Developmental delay
  - Relapse or recurrence: may occur despite treatment with acyclovir. May require long-term treatment with antiviral agents for months.

INTRAUTERINE INFECTIONS

Intrauterine infections may cause damage to the developing nervous system, including hydrocephalus, cerebral atrophy, intracranial calcifications, and hydranencephaly. Postnatally, these features are associated with retardation, long tract signs, seizures, microcephaly, hearing loss, chorioretinitis, and hydrocephalus.

Systemic signs appearing postnatally that are associated with intrauterine infections are hepatomegaly, small for gestational age, rash, petechiae, and jaundice. Intrauterine infections are classically grouped under the acronym TORCH as follows: toxoplasmosis, rubella, cytomegalic virus, herpes simplex, human immunodeficiency virus (HIV) (newly included) (Table 16.2).

Acute Disseminated Encephalomyelitis

Clinical Features

- Monophasic demyelinating disease of the nervous system
- Usually follows respiratory infection; occurs days to several weeks after urinary tract infection
- Winter and spring distribution
- Associated with the subsequent development of multiple sclerosis rarely
- Etiologic agent rarely recovered

Course

- Acute neurologic deterioration seen
- May need respiratory support
- Recovery not directly related to severity of neurologic damage

- Most: recovery with no or limited deficit.
- Treatment: mainly supportive; consists of steroids, intravenous immunoglobulin (Ig) (both have limited effectiveness)

Imaging

- Multifocal T2 and flair lesions: independent of clinical course
- Involves subcortical white matter, brainstem, and spinal cord
- T1 lesions: less pronounced
- Gradual resolution of MRI changes over many months: unrelated to clinical recovery.

TORCH Infections

As was stated above, TORCH infection is an acronym for a group of congenital infections occurring in the intrauterine and perinatal period of time. Toxoplasmosis, cytomegalovirus, and herpes virus, type II, are the classical TORCH infections. Increasingly, neonatal HIV should be considered as part of the TORCH spectrum.

Neonatal Toxoplasmosis

Clinical Features

- Chorioretinitis
- Hydrocephalus
- Intracranial calcification
  - Periventricular
  - Basal ganglia
  - Cerebral parenchyma

Diagnosis

- Antitoxoplasma IgM: peaks at 2 weeks
- Antitoxoplasma IgG: peaks at 0 to 8 weeks

Treatment

- Pyrimethamine
- Sulfadiazine

Neonatal Cytomegalovirus

Clinical Features

- Chorioretinitis
- Hydrocephalus
- Intracranial calcification—more diffuse than in toxoplasmosis
- Hearing loss

- Microcephaly
- Hepatosplenomegaly

Diagnosis

- Virus shed in urine
- PCR of urine, saliva, or serum

Treatment

Ganciclovir is used to treat neonatal cytomegalic virus.

Rubella

Clinical Features

- Cataracts
- Congenital heart disease
- Hearing loss
- Microcephaly
- Hepatosplenomegaly
- Intrauterine growth retardation

Diagnosis

- Isolate virus from urine; also seen in nasopharynx
- PCR for virus

Treatment

Treatment consists of vaccinating all expectant mothers.

Neonatal Herpes (Most Often Type II)

Clinical Features

- Vertical transmission
- Seizures
- Lethargy
- Microcephaly
- Cataracts
- Intracranial calcification
- Rash
- Multiorgan involvement

Diagnosis

- Isolate virus from CSF
- PCR

- MRI: diffuse changes differ from older age onset herpes, which are usually located in the temporal lobes.

Treatment

Give acyclovir, 20 mg per kg, three times a day for 21 days.

Neonatal Human Immunodeficiency Virus

Clinical Features

- Vertical transmission
- May not become symptomatic until third month of life
- Hepatomegaly
- Rash
- Failure to thrive
- Microcephaly

Diagnosis

- PCR
- P24 antigen detection
- Abnormal imaging
  - Calcification of basal ganglia
  - Cortical atrophy
- Brain directly invaded
- Opportunistic infection: less common than adults
- Lymphoma: rare in children

Treatment

- Multidrug treatment to reduce viral load
- Zidovudine therapy of HIV-infected mothers

BRAIN ABSCESS

Brain abscess is defined as a localized collection of pus within the parenchyma of the brain.

Origin

- Paranasal sinuses
  - Frontal sinuses not developed in children until 9 to 10 years of age
  - Seen after trauma or surgery
  - Complication of otitis media

- Hematogenous
  - Cyanotic heart disease
  - Patent foramen ovale
  - Pulmonary infection
- Immune deficiencies
- Bacterial endocarditis

Etiology

- *Staphylococcus aureus*
- Anaerobic streptococcus
- Anaerobic gram-negative rods
- Mixed flora

Clinical Features

- Seizures
- Subtle long tract signs
- Increased intracranial pressure
- Absent to low grade fever; high fever suggests rupture of abscess wall with passage of pyrogens into the bloodstream
- Abscess: stage of cerebritis, followed by the development of a capsular wall
  - Capsule formation occurs 10 days to weeks after the exciting organism initially invades the brain.
  - Search for a history of chronic infection or past infection.
- Imaging: computed tomography or MRI is diagnostic
  - Computed tomography shows hypodense core with enhancing rim.
  - MRI shows increased T1 hypointense core with enhancing rim.
  - T2 shows increased signal intensity of core with evidence of capsule formation.

Treatment

- Management of increased intracranial pressure
- Surgical drainage
- Antibiotics
  - Begin with 4 to 6 weeks of antibiotics. May preclude surgery.
  - Use broad-spectrum antibiotics, such as metronidazole, cefotaxime, and vancomycin.
  - If possible, obtain culture before therapy.

- Repeat MRI every 2 to 3 months after either antibiotics or surgical drainage to visualize the collapse of abscess and the regression of the abscess cavity.

Suggested Reading

Ashwal S, Perkin RM, Thompson JR, et al. Bacterial meningitis in children: current concepts of neurologic management. *Curr Probl Pediatr* 1996;24:267–284.

Peter G, ed. *Red book: report on the Committee on Infectious Diseases.* Elk Grove, IL: American Academy of Pediatrics, 2000.

Tyler KL, Martin JB. *Infectious diseases of the central nervous system.* Philadelphia: FA Davis, 1993. Contemporary Neurology Series.

Chapter 17

Seizures

Case

A 6-year-old child presents to the emergency room with a complaint of inattentiveness and staring spells. She is unaware of these episodes. No aura or postictal state is seen. The teacher complains that, in a day, the child has many of these daydreaming episodes lasting a few seconds each. Her school performance has been erratic, which seems to correlate with the frequency of the staring spells. The child's past medical history is unremarkable. She has no history of head trauma. No family history of seizures is present. The child's neurologic examination is normal. Hyperventilation produces a 3-second staring spell unaccompanied by aura or postictal confusion. An electroencephalogram (EEG) shows a 3-Hz spike and wave pattern in a generalized distribution activated by hyperventilation.

Diagnosis

Absence seizures
She was placed on valproic acid with complete resolution of symptomatology.

The definition of seizure is an excessive and disorderly discharge of nervous tissue, the manifestations of which depend on where in the brain the discharges arise and to where they spread. **Epilepsy** is defined as more than one unprovoked seizure.

GENERALIZED SEIZURES

- These begin centrally in the nonspecific nuclei of thalamus and spread bilaterally and synchronously to all parts of the nervous system.
- A loss of consciousness *always* occurs.
- If a motor component is present, it is always symmetric.
- The prognosis varies with age at onset.

Infantile Spasms

- Ninety percent begin in the first year of life; the peak age of onset is 4 to 6 months of age.
- Infantile spasms syndrome (West syndrome) is defined by the following:
  - Jack-knife seizures (myoclonic) in clusters
  - Hypsarrhythmic EEG
  - Mental retardation (behavioral regression)

Etiology

- Cryptogenic (unknown): previously normal child
- Symptomatic (anything that damages the developing nervous system)
  - Etiology in more than 75%
  - Tuberous sclerosis in 20% of cases
  - Central nervous system malformations (e.g., Aicardi syndrome, consisting of agenesis corpus callosum, retinal lacunae, infantile spasms and seen only in females; heterotopias)
  - Metabolic disorders
  - Birth asphyxia
  - Brain tumor
  - Meningitis

Evaluation

- Skin: view with ultraviolet light to identify ash-leaf spots (nevus anemicus), which are associated with tuberous sclerosis
- EEG
  - Typical hypsarrhythmic pattern: chaotic high voltage spikes, sharp waves; no normal background; burst suppression may or may not be present

    - Modified hypsarrhythmia with some normal background in 40%
    - Periodicity during sleep and ictally
- Magnetic resonance imaging (MRI): shows congenital malformations
- Blood and urine amino acids (AA); urine organic acids, ammonia, lactate, pyruvate, and biotinidase
    - Pyridoxine trial (give pyridoxine, 50 to 100 mg intravenously, during EEG monitoring)
    - Ophthalmologic examination
        - Chorioretinal lacunas (Aicardi syndrome)
        - Cherry red spot (Tay-Sachs, metachromatic leukodystrophy [MLD])
        - Chorioretinitis (congenital infection)
        - Optic atrophy (Krabbe disease, MLD)

Treatment

- First choice: adrenocorticotropic hormone (ACTH) or prednisone
- Other (not in rank order): clonazepam, primidone, vigabitrine (not approved in the United States but drug of choice for patients with tuberous sclerosis in Europe)

Prognosis

- Cryptogenic: 30% have normal intelligence
- Symptomatic: 10% have normal intelligence, 50% develop other seizures

Myoclonic Epilepsies of Early Childhood

- Onset occurs from 12 months to 5 years of age.
- Myoclonic, akinetic, and absence seizures occur many times a day.
- EEG shows polyspike and waves that are generalized.
- These types of seizures are difficult to control.
- The prognosis is generally poor, although some patients resolve without sequelae.

Evaluation

- EEG
- Metabolic evaluation
- MRI of the brain

Treatment

(Not in rank order)

- Clonazepam
- Ethosuximide
- Lamotrigine
- Topiramate
- Valproic acid
- Ketogenic diet

Lennox-Gastaut Syndrome

Clinical

- Appears from 1 to 6 years of age
- Tonic, atonic, myoclonic, and atypical absence seizures; episodes of nonconvulsive status epilepticus
- Frequent daily seizures
- Mental retardation: progressive
- EEG
  - Slow spike and wave
  - Activated during drowsiness and slow sleep

Etiologies

- Neurocutaneous syndromes
  - Tuberous sclerosis
  - Linear nevus sebaceous
- Leigh disease
- Perinatal insult
- Aminoacidopathies
- Storage disease
- Neuronal ceroid lipofuscinosis

Evaluation

- MRI
- Metabolic evaluation
- Consider rectal, skin, and conjunctival biopsies

Treatment

Treatment is usually ineffective; however, the following (not in rank order) may be used:

- Possibly corticotropin
- Clonazepam
- Felbamate
- Lamotrigine
- Topiramate
- Valproic acid
- Ketogenic diet

Prognosis

The prognosis is poor. The following long-term residua are seen:

- Epilepsy
- Mental retardation

Absence Seizures

- Age of onset: 3 to 12 years
- Aura: none
- Postictal state: none
- Clinical symptoms: staring, eye blinking, loss of consciousness
- Duration: seconds
- Frequency: many in a day
- EEG: 3-Hz spike and wave (generalized)
- Etiology: genetic

Evaluation

The EEG is used for evaluation.

- Activated by hyperventilation
- Often activated by photic stimulation
- MRI and computed tomography not indicated

Treatment

- First choice: ethosuximide or valproic acid
- Others (not in rank order): acetazolamide, clonazepam, lamotrigine

The prognosis with treatment is good, and these usually resolve in adolescence.

Generalized Tonic-Clonic Seizures

- Age of onset can be any time beyond the neonatal period until senescence.

- No aura is present (aura suggests secondary generalized tonic-clonic seizure with focal cortical onset).
- Tonic stiffening, loss of consciousness, apnea, with or without bladder or bowel incontinence and tongue biting, are seen.
- After these, the following occur:
  - Clonic activity in four limbs: symmetric
  - Postictal confusion or sleep
  - Recovery

Evaluation

- EEG: in the interictal period, bilateral epileptiform discharges are seen.
- Imaging if history suggests a focal onset, the examination is abnormal, or the EEG is focal

Treatment

Options for treatment include the following (not in rank order):

- Carbamazepine (if no spike-wave pattern is seen)
- Gabapentin
- Lamotrigine
- Phenobarbital
- Phenytoin
- Topiramate
- Valproic acid (if older than 3 years of age)

Juvenile Myoclonic Epilepsy

- Age of onset: 8 to 24 years
- Family history: positive
- Gender: females have this far more often than males
- Normal examination, normal intelligence
- Myoclonic seizures: occur in early morning
- Generalized tonic-clonic seizures: occur during sleep
- May also have absence seizures
- EEG: 3.5-Hz to 6-Hz spike and wave, polyspike and wave (generalized)
- MRI and computed tomography: not indicated if the history and EEG are typical
- Treatment (not in rank order): lamotrigine, valproic acid
- May be exacerbated by sleep deprivation and alcohol
- Relapse: 90% after cessation of medication

SEIZURES BEGINNING LOCALLY

Partial Seizures (Three Types)

- Simple (without impaired consciousness)
- Complex (with impaired consciousness)
- Secondarily generalized (simple or complex spreading to bilateral involvement)

Features of Simple Partial Seizures (Focal Motor or Focal Sensory)

- Seen at any age
- Little or no warning
- Focal limb movement (focal motor) *or* sequential muscle contractions (Jacksonian seizure) *or* focal numbness, burning, or tingling (focal sensory)
- No loss of consciousness
- No postictal confusion but may have Todd paralysis; neuronal exhaustion phenomenon; transient focal weakness
- MRI: rule out structural lesion
- EEG: focal spikes or sharp waves in 40% to 85% of patients

Treatment

The following may be used for treatment of partial seizures (not in rank order):

- Carbamazepine
- Gabapentin
- Lamotrigine
- Levetiracetam
- Oxcarbazepine
- Phenytoin
- Topiramate
- Valproic acid
- Zonisamide

Benign Rolandic Epilepsy

Clinical Features

- Most common partial epilepsy in childhood
- Begins from 2 to 12 years of age (usually between the ages of 5 to 10); ends by early adolescence
- Nocturnal: secondarily generalized tonic-clonic seizures

- Diurnal: partial seizures
  - Orobuccal movements or sensation, drooling
  - Speech arrest
- EEG: spike or spike and wave in the midtemporal and central sylvian (rolandic) regions with phase reversals; may be unilateral or bilateral
- Positive family history of abnormal EEGs (autosomal dominant); only 12% have seizures
- Evaluation
  - EEG: first choice
  - MRI: obtain if neurologic examination is abnormal or EEG is not typical or focal

Treatment

The following (not in rank order) constitute the available therapies:

- Carbamazepine (treat for 1 to 2 years) or no treatment (many have only one or two seizures)
- Gabapentin
- Lamotrigine
- Levetiracetam
- Oxcarbazepine
- Phenytoin
- Topiramate
- Valproic acid
- Zonisamide

Benign Occipital Epilepsy of Childhood

- Simple partial seizures with predominantly visual symptoms (colors and shapes) occur.
- Spike and/or slow wave activity occurs over one or both occipital areas. Activity is arrested or decreased by eye opening.
- Generally, the prognosis is good.

Gelastic Seizures

- Begin in children younger than 2 years of age
- "Giggling"
- Associated with hamartomas of the hypothalamus; precocious puberty—frequent
- Evolve into secondarily generalized seizures

Complex Partial Seizures With Impaired Consciousness

Clinical Features

- Onset at any age
- Aura: present
  - Upset stomach or nausea
  - Urgent need to defecate
  - Unpleasant smells or tastes
  - Auditory or visual hallucinations
  - Depersonalization
  - Intense fear
  - Déjà vu
  - Jamais vu
- Staring with automatisms (playing with hair, lip smacking, picking at clothing, nonsense speech)
- Duration: 1 to 2 minutes (more or less)
- Frequency: one to two times per day or less
- Postictal state: present; consists of confusion and sleep
- EEG: temporal sharp waves and rhythmic temporal theta or alpha
- Etiology: may be structural
- Obtain MRI (computed tomography does not provide adequate view of temporal lobes)
  - Tumor
  - Mesial temporal sclerosis
  - Dysplasia

Treatment

The following may be used for treatment (not in rank order):

- Carbamazepine
- Gabapentin
- Lamotrigine
- Levetiracetam
- Oxcarbazepine
- Phenobarbital
- Phenytoin
- Primidone
- Tiagibine
- Topiramate
- Valproic acid
- Zonisamide

TABLE 17.1 Timetable for the Treatment of Status Epilepticus

Time (Min)	Drug and Nondrug Treatment
0	Ensure adequate respiration; intubation may be necessary, and low flow oxygen should be started.
2–3	Start i.v. with normal saline. First, draw blood for anticonvulsant levels, glucose, hepatic and renal functions, CBC with differential, electrolytes, Ca, Mg, blood gases and toxicology screen. Obtain urine for routine U/A.
5	Start second i.v. line. Give lorazepam, 4 mg (0.1 mg/kg), or diazepam, 10 mg (0.2 mg/kg)—infuse i.v. over 2 min with saline for simultaneous administration of second medication and i.v. fluids.
7–8	Administer phenytoin or fosphenytoin, 20 mg/kg (between 1,000 and 2,000 mg in most adults), i.v. push. Dilute in saline and infuse at a rate of no more than 0.75 mg/kg of body weight (no more than 50 mg/min of phenytoin or 150 mg/min of phenytoin equivalents of fosphenytoin in adults). In children less than 18 mo of age, give pyridoxine, 100–200 mg i.v. Monitor EKG and blood pressure.
10	Administer a benzodiazepine; may be repeated.
30–60	Start continuous EEG monitoring, unless status has stopped and the patient is waking up.
40	Give phenobarbital, 20 mg/kg (between 1,000 and 2,000 mg in most adults). Dilute in saline and infuse at a rate of no more than 0.75 mg/min/kg of body weight (50 mg/min in adults).
70	Administer pentobarbital; load with 3–5 mg/kg given over 3–5 min. Then start continuous infusion at 1 mg/kg/h; increase continuous infusion with additional smaller loading doses until EEG burst and/or suppression. (Alternative is midazolam at a loading dose of 0.15–0.20 mg/kg, followed by infusion of 0.05–0.30 mg/kg/h. EEG should be monitored and infusion should be stopped, at least temporarily, after 12 h to check for seizure recurrence.)

Abbreviations: Ca, calcium; CBC, complete blood count; EEG, electroencephalogram; EKG, electrocardiogram; i.v., intravenous; Mg, magnesium; U/A, urinanalysis.

Modified from the American Epilepsy Society. Medical education program residents version. *Clinical epilepsy*, slides 38 and 39. West Hartford, CT: American Epilepsy Society, 1999. Available at: http://www.aesnet.org/ppt/clinical/index.cfm. Accessed January 23, 2003, with permission.

Partial Seizures with Secondary Generalization

This consists of seizures that begin focally in the cortex and then spread to the nonspecific nuclei of the thalamus, with secondary excitation of both cerebral hemispheres.

TABLE 17.2 Indications Approved by the Food and Drug Administration for the Newer Anticonvulsants

Drug	Indications
Gabapentin	Adjunctive therapy in treatment of partial seizures with and without secondary generalization in patients over 12 yr of age Adjunctive therapy in treatment of partial seizures in pediatric patients from 3–12 yr of age
Lamotrigine	Monotherapy use: adults over 16 yr of age with partial seizures who had been taking a single enzyme-inducing antiepileptic drug (EIAED) Adjunctive use: adult patients with partial seizures with and without secondary generalization With pediatric and adult patients in treatment of generalized seizures of Lennox-Gastaut syndrome
Levetiracetam	Adjunctive therapy in adults over 16 yr of age in treatment of partial onset seizures
Oxcarbazepine	Monotherapy use: adults (individuals older than 16 yr of age) in treatment of partial seizures Adjunctive use: adults and children from 4 to 16 yr of age in treatment of partial seizures
Tiagibine	Adjunctive therapy in adults and children over 12 yr of age with partial seizures
Topiramate	Adjunctive therapy in adults and pediatric patients 2 yr of age and older with partial onset seizures or primary generalized tonic-clonic seizures and in patients over 2 yr of age with Lennox-Gastaut syndrome
Zonisamide	Adjunctive therapy in treatment of partial seizures in adults older than 16 yr of age

History

- Aura may be present, suggesting a cortical onset.
- Seizure begins with a focal onset.

Examination

The examination may reveal the following focal findings in the postictal period (e.g., unilateral Babinski, Todd paralysis).

Evaluation

- EEG: focal discharges with secondary generalization
- MRI

Treatment

The following may be used for treatment of partial seizures with secondary generalization (not in rank order):

- Carbamazepine
- Gabapentin
- Lamotrigine
- Levetiracetam
- Oxcarbazepine
- Tiagibine
- Topiramate
- Valproic acid
- Zonisamide

ADDITIONAL RESOURCES

See Table 17.1 for the American Epilepsy Society recommendations for treatment of status epilepticus. In addition, United States Food and Drug Administration-approved indications for the newer anticonvulsants are listed in Table 17.2.

Suggested Reading

Aicardi J. *Epilepsy in children.* New York: Raven Press, 1986.

Annegers JF, Shirts SB, Hauser WA, et al. Risk of recurrence after an initial unprovoked seizure. *Epilepsia* 1986;27:43–50.

Boulloche J, Leloup P, Mallet E, et al. Risk of recurrence after a single unprovoked, generalized tonic-clonic seizure. *Dev Med Child Neurol* 1989;31:626–632.

Bouma PA, Peters AC, Arts RJ, et al. Discontinuation of antiepileptic therapy: a prospective study in children. *J Neurol Neurosurg Psychiatry* 1987; 50:1579–1583.

Cowan LD, Hudson LS. The epidemiology and natural history of infantile spasms. *J Child Neurol* 1991;6:355–364.

Delgado-Escueta AV, Enrile-Bascal FE. Juvenile myoclonic epilepsy of Janz. *Neurology* 1984;34:285–294.

Devinsky O, Kelley K. Porter RJ, et al. Clinical and electro-encephalographic features of simple partial seizures. *Neurology* 1988;38:1347–1352.

Donat J. The age-dependent epileptic encephalopathies. *J Child Neurol* 1992;7:7–21.

Dulac O, Chugani HT, Dalla Bernadina B. *Infantile spasms and West syndrome.* Philadelphia: WB Saunders, 1994.

Ferrendelli JA. Juvenile myoclonic epilepsy. *Epilepsia* 1989;30:S1–S27.

Frank LM, Enlow T, Holmes GL. Lamictal (Lamotrigine) monotherapy for typical absence seizures in children. *Epilepsia* 1999;40:973–979.

Hirtz D, Ashwal S, Berg A, et al. Practice parameter: evaluating a first non-febrile seizure in children. Report of the Quality Standards Subcommittee of the American Academy of Neurology, the Child Neurology Society, and the American Epilepsy Society. *Neurology* 2000;55:616–623.

Holmes GL. *Diagnosis and management of seizures in children.* Philadelphia: WB Saunders, 1987.

Holmes GL. Myoclonic, tonic, and atonic seizures in children. *J Epilepsy* 1988;1:173–195.

Holmes GL. Partial seizures in children. *Pediatrics* 1986;77:725–731.

Holmes GL. Surgery for intractable seizures in infants and early childhood. *Neurology* 1993;43:S28–S37.

Holmes GL, McKeever M, Adamson M. Absence seizures in children: clinical and electroencephalographic features. *Ann Neurol* 1987;21: 268–273.

Kotagal P, Rothner AD, Erenberg G, et al. Complex partial seizures of childhood onset. *Arch Neurol* 1987;44:1177–1180.

Loiseau P, Duche B, Cordova S, et al. Prognosis of benign childhood epilepsy with centrotemporal spikes: a follow-up study of 168 patients. *Epilepsia* 1988;29:229–235.

Markand ON. Slow spike-wave activity in EEG and associated clinical features: often called "Lennox" or "Lennox-Gastaut" syndrome. *Neurology* 1977;27:746–757.

Motte J, Trevathan E, Arvidsson JF, et al. Lamotrigine for generalized seizures associated with the Lennox-Gastaut syndrome. *N Engl J Med* 1997;337:1807–1812.

Panayiotopoulos CP. Benign childhood epilepsy with occipital paroxysms: a 15-year prospective study. *Ann Neurol* 1989;26:51–56.

Panayiotopoulos CP. Benign nocturnal childhood occipital epilepsy: a new syndrome with nocturnal seizures, tonic deviation of the eyes and vomiting. *J Child Neurol* 1989;4:43–48.

Shinnar S, Berg AT, Moshé SL, et al. Discontinuing antiepileptic drugs in children with epilepsy: a prospective study. *Ann Neurol* 1994;35:534–545.

Shinnar S, Berg AT, Moshé S. Risk of seizure recurrence following unprovoked seizure in childhood: a prospective study. *Pediatrics* 1990;85: 1076–1085.

Shinnar S, Vining EP, Mellits ED, et al. Discontinuing antiepileptic medication in children with epilepsy after two years without seizures. *N Engl J Med* 1985;313:976–980.

Snead OC. Treatment of infantile spasms. *Pediatr Neurol* 1990;6:147–150.

Treatment of convulsive status epilepticus. Recommendations of the Epilepsy Foundation of America's Working Group on Status Epilepticus. *JAMA* 1993;270:854–859.

Wyllie E, Rothner AD, Lüders H. Partial seizures in children: clinical features, medical treatment, and surgical considerations. *Pediatr Clin North Am* 1989;36:343–364.

Zupanc ML, Handler EG, Levinc RL, et al. Rasmussen encephalitis: epilepsia partialis continua secondary to chronic encephalitis. *Pediatr Neurol* 1990;6:397–401.

Chapter 18

Febrile Seizures

Case

A 2-year-old child presents to the emergency room with a first generalized tonic-clonic seizure lasting 2 minutes. On arrival, the child is alert, but he has a fever of 39.9°C (103.8°F). He has no meningismus. The neurologic examination is normal. The general examination reveals bilateral otitis media. His past medical history and development are normal. The father has a positive family history of febrile seizures.

Diagnosis

Simple febrile seizures

Febrile seizures occur in 2% to 4% of children. They are divided into the following two types: simple and complex. By definition, they occur in febrile children from 6 months to 5 years of age who do not have a central nervous system infection. Complex and simple febrile seizures differ in length, description, and the number of seizures in 24 hours. A positive family history is common.

CHARACTERISTICS OF FEBRILE SEIZURES

Simple Febrile Seizures

- Generalized tonic-clonic seizure **plus**
- No more than 15 minutes duration **plus**
- One seizure in 24 hours

Complex Febrile Seizures

- Focal (partial) seizure *or*
- More than 15 minutes duration *or*
- Flurry (more than one seizure in 24 hours)

Recurrence Rate

- First simple febrile seizure before 12 months of age: 50% recur
- First simple febrile seizure after 12 months of age: 30% recur
- Two or more febrile seizures: 50% recur

NEURODIAGNOSTIC EVALUATION OF THE CHILD WITH A FIRST *SIMPLE* FEBRILE SEIZURE

The following is according to the American Academy of Pediatrics practice parameter.

- Evaluate the source of the fever
- Consider lumbar puncture
  - Strongly, if younger than 12 months of age
  - At 12 to 18 months of age, use clinical judgment
  - With clinical suspicion, if more than 18 months of age
- Further evaluation of seizure (i.e., electroencephalogram, blood studies, neuroimaging) usually not required

LONG-TERM TREATMENT OF THE CHILD WITH SIMPLE FEBRILE SEIZURES

The following is according to the American Academy of Pediatrics Practice parameter. The theoretical risks of *simple* febrile seizures are as follows:

- Risk of epilepsy: 2.4% by 25 years of age if the child is neurologically normal. No evidence indicates that simple febrile seizures cause structural disease or that treatment prevents epilepsy.
- Adverse effects on cognition: no adverse effects on cognition have been identified.
- Premature death: no cases of premature death with simple febrile seizures have been reported.
- Risk of recurrence: 50% if the first seizure is before 12 months of age; 30% if the first seizure is after 12 months of age; and 50% risk of recurrence thereafter.

Can Recurrent Simple Febrile Seizures Be Prevented with Continuous Anticonvulsant Therapy?

- Phenobarbital: prevents 90% of recurrences if level is therapeutic
- Phenytoin and carbamazepine: ineffective
- Valproic acid: significantly better than the placebo; at least as effective as phenobarbital

Can Recurrent Simple Febrile Seizures Be Prevented with Intermittent Therapy?

- Acetaminophen: acetaminophen does not prevent recurrent simple febrile seizures when used alone.
- Diazepam: intermittent oral diazepam (0.33 mg per kg every 8 hours for 48 hours) will significantly reduce the risk of recurrences.

What are the Risks of Anticonvulsant Therapy?

- Phenobarbital: 20% to 45% of patients have behavioral disturbances and hyperactivity.
- Valproic acid: fatal hepatotoxicity, thrombocytopenia, pancreatitis, and weight loss or weight gain can occur.
- Diazepam: ataxia, lethargy, irritability, sleep disorders, and the potential to mask central nervous system infection are seen.

RECOMMENDATIONS OF THE AMERICAN ACADEMY OF PEDIATRICS

Based on the risks and benefits of the effective therapies, neither continuous nor intermittent anticonvulsant therapy is recommended for children with one or more *simple* febrile seizures.

COMPLEX FEBRILE SEIZURES

Definition

- Occur from 6 months to 5 years of age
- Fever
- No central nervous system infection
- Seizure more than 15 minutes *or* partial *or* more than 1 in 24 hours

Risk of Epilepsy

- Risk of temporal lobe epilepsy by 25 years of age is 49% if all three characteristics—prolonged, partial, and flurry—are present.
- The following two theories have been formulated for why the risk of epilepsy is so high:
  - The prolonged partial febrile seizure may cause mesial temporal sclerosis, leading to a focus for temporal lobe epilepsy.
  - The patient has underlying mesial temporal sclerosis (possibly that is perinatal in origin), which acts as focus for complex febrile seizures and later for temporal lobe epilepsy.

Evaluation

- Lumbar puncture: higher incidence of meningitis with complex febrile seizures than with simple febrile seizures.
- Consider magnetic resonance imaging, especially if a partial seizure occurs; assess for mesial temporal sclerosis and other structural lesions

Treatment

- Administer rectal diazepam for prolonged seizures.
- Consider prophylaxis, such as phenobarbital.

No American Academy of Pediatrics practice parameter for complex febrile seizures is available at this time.

Suggested Reading

American Academy of Pediatrics Committee on Quality Improvement, Subcommittee on Febrile Seizures. Practice parameter: long-term treatment of the child with simple febrile seizures. *Pediatrics* 1999; 103:1307–1309.

American Academy of Pediatrics Provisional Committee on Quality Improvement, Subcommittee on Febrile Seizures. Practice parameter: the neurodiagnostic evaluation of the child with a first simple febrile seizure. *Pediatrics* 1996;97:769–775.

Annegers JF, Hauser WA, Shirts SB, et al. Factors prognostic of unprovoked seizures after febrile convulsions. *N Engl J Med* 1987;316: 493–498.

Baumann RJ, Duffner PK. Treatment of children with simple febrile seizures: the AAP practice parameter [Review]. *Pediatr Neurol* 2000; 23:11–17.

Camfield PR, Camfield CS, Shapiro SH, et al. The first febrile seizure: antipyretic instruction plus either phenobarbital or placebo to prevent recurrence. *J Pediatr* 1980;97:16–21.

Ellenberg JH, Nelson KB. Febrile seizures and later intellectual performance. *Arch Neurol* 1978;35:17–21.

Nelson KB, Ellenberg JH. Predictors of epilepsy in children who have experienced febrile seizures. *N Engl J Med* 1976;295:1029–1033.

Chapter 19

Neonatal Seizures

Case

A newborn infant began having tonic seizures 16 hours after birth. Delivery had been complicated by a depressed fetal heart rate and an emergency cesarean section. At birth, the child was hypotonic and apneic, requiring resuscitation. Apgar scores were 0 at 1 minute and 2 at 5 minutes. On examination, the child was extremely hypotonic with a poor cry and absent neonatal reflexes. The seizures were treated with 20 mg per kg of intravenous phenobarbital. The seizures stopped within 24 hours. A computed tomography scan showed evidence of diffuse hypodensity with cerebral edema, and the electroencephalogram (EEG) showed multifocal sharp waves with suppressed background. The child gradually improved, and the EEG normalized. Phenobarbital was discontinued before discharge at 3 weeks of age.

Diagnosis

Neonatal seizures secondary to hypoxic-ischemic encephalopathy

TYPES

- Subtle
  - Sucking
  - Abnormal posture
  - Peddling
  - Nystagmus

- Apnea
- Autonomic (flushing, cyanosis)
- Clonic: focal
- Clonic: multifocal
- Myoclonic
- Generalized tonic
- Nonepileptic seizures
  - Stimulus sensitive
  - Suppressed with passive restraint
  - Not accompanied by autonomic changes

ETIOLOGY

First Three Days

- Hypoxic-ischemic encephalopathy
  - Ninety percent of seizures: days 1 and 2
  - Almost always secondary to an intrauterine event, such as partial prolonged asphyxia
- Hemorrhage: intraventricular, subarachnoid, or subdural
- Trauma
- Metabolic: decreased blood sugar (especially small for gestational age); decreased calcium, magnesium, or sodium; sodium may also be increased
- Pyridoxine dependency
- Nonketotic hyperglycinemia
- Local anesthetic intoxication
- Sepsis and meningitis

Late Onset: After Three Days

- Hemorrhage
- Meningitis: group B hemolytic streptococci, *Escherichia coli, Listeria monocytogenes*
- Viral encephalitis: toxoplasmosis, herpes, cytomegalovirus, adenovirus, influenza
- Metabolic: amino acids, organic acids
- Primary hypocalcemia and hypomagnesemia: dietary; immature renal and parathyroid function
- Drug withdrawal
- Brain anomalies
- Fifth-day fits

- ◆ Days 4 to 6: healthy full-term infants
- ◆ Seizures severe for 24 hours, then resolve; usually stop by the end of week 2
- ◆ Good prognosis

- ■ Benign neonatal sleep myoclonus (nonepileptic)
  - ◆ Synchronous bilateral clonic activity during the early stages of sleep
  - ◆ EEG: normal or sharp transients
  - ◆ Seizures stop when child is awakened; do not stop with restraint unless awakened
  - ◆ Treatment not indicated
  - ◆ Good prognosis
- ■ Benign familial neonatal seizures
  - ◆ Autosomal dominant: chromosome 20.8q
  - ◆ Persist for 1 to 6 months
  - ◆ Normal development; approximately 15% risk of epilepsy

EVALUATION

- ■ Take history and conduct physical examination.
- ■ The following tests should be performed routinely:
  - ◆ Blood sugar, calcium, magnesium, sodium, blood urea nitrogen, creatinine, total carbon dioxide (TCO_2), ammonia, bilirubin
  - ◆ Blood gas and urine ketones
  - ◆ Drug screen
  - ◆ Lumbar puncture
  - ◆ Cultures: bacterial and viral
  - ◆ Pyridoxine trial: give 50 to 100 mg intravenously during EEG monitoring
  - ◆ EEG
  - ◆ Computed tomography and magnetic resonance imaging
- ■ The following should be performed if the diagnosis is obscure:
  - ◆ Blood and urine amino acids
  - ◆ Urine organic acids
  - ◆ Cerebrospinal fluid glycine (nonketotic hyperglycinemia)
  - ◆ Blood and/or cerebrospinal fluid lactate and pyruvate (mitochondrial disease, organic acidurias)
  - ◆ Very long chain fatty acids (neonatal adrenoleukodystrophy)
  - ◆ Lysosomal enzymes

TREATMENT

Acute

- Phenobarbital, 20 mg per kg intravenously. If seizure persists, increase to 40 mg per kg (serum levels of 20 to 40 μg per mL)
- Seizure continues: give phenytoin, 10 mg per kg intravenously; repeat once, up to 20 mg per kg (not to exceed 1 mg per kg per min; levels of 15 to 20 μg per mL)
- Seizure still continues: administer diazepam, 0.1 mg per kg intravenously, or lorazepam, 0.05 mg per kg intravenously

Maintenance

- Phenobarbital: levels more than 15 μg per mL
- Discontinuation of anticonvulsants in neonatal period with low-risk patients: 2 weeks after last seizure and no electrographic seizures on EEG

Suggested Reading

Holmes GL. Neonatal seizures. *Semin Pediatr Neurol* 1994;1:72–82.

Leppert M, Anderson VE, Quattelbaum T, et al. Benign familial neonatal convulsions linked to genetic markers on chromosome 20. *Nature* 1989;337:647–648.

Mizrahi EM, Kellaway P. Characterization and classification of neonatal seizures. *Neurology* 1987;37:1837–1844.

Volpe JJ. *Neurology of the newborn,* 3rd ed. Philadelphia: WB Saunders, 1995.

Chapter 20

Nonepileptic Paroxysmal Events

Case

A 13-year-old girl "passed out" in church. The day was warm, and she had been kneeling. When she stood up, she felt light-headed, diaphoretic, and nauseated, and her vision became dark. She then lost consciousness and slumped to the ground. The spell lasted 2 minutes, after which she was embarrassed, but had no sequelae. She had no history of cardiac disease or seizures.

Diagnosis

Vasovagal syncope

SYNCOPE

Syncope is defined as a transient loss of consciousness and posture from inadequate cerebral perfusion (Table 20.1).

Etiology

Vasovagal

- Begins with a light-headed sensation, nausea, clouding of vision, or the constriction of visual fields and is followed by slumping or falling to the ground with a loss of consciousness
- Can occur with or without incontinence
- Skin: pale, cold, and clammy
- Pulse: slow
- Tonic-clonic activity: may follow at times

TABLE 20.1 Comparison of Syncope and Seizures

	Syncope	Seizure
Position related	Upright, usually standing	–
Aura	Prolonged	±
Color	Pallor	Rubor or cyanosis or normal
Tone	Limp	Tonic
Incontinence	Rare	Frequent
Postictal	Rare	Common
Injury	Rare	±
Abnormal EEG	Rare	Common

Abbreviation: EEG, electroencephalogram.

- Occurs in upright, usually standing position
- Positive family history: typical

Cardiac Origin

- Arrhythmias
  - Prolonged QT interval
  - Wolff–Parkinson–White syndrome
  - Sick sinus syndrome
- Decreased cardiac output
  - Aortic stenosis
  - Cardiomyopathy

Cerebrovascular

This etiology is uncommon in children.

- Carotid disease
- Vertebrobasilar disease

Metabolic

- Hypoglycemia
- Anemia
  - Bleeding
  - Hemoglobinopathy
  - Hemolytic disease
  - Iron deficiency
- Decreased partial pressure of carbon dioxide (P_{CO_2}) secondary to hyperventilation

Evaluation

- Blood sugar, complete blood count
- Electrocardiogram, Holter tape
- Chest x-ray
- Echocardiogram
- Tilt table—helpful for neurocardiogenic syncope and postural orthostatic tachycardia syndrome
- Electroencephalogram: may or may not be indicated, depending on history
- Magnetic resonance imaging: may or may not be needed, depending on history and examination

BREATH-HOLDING SPELLS

Cyanotic Type

- Onset rarely seen after 24 months of age; peak at 12 months (0 to 18 months); gone by 4 to 6 years of age
- Provoked by fear, anger, and/or pain
- Clinical features
  - Child cries; becomes apneic in expiration; leads to cyanosis
  - Loss of consciousness seen
  - Becomes limp
  - Brief stiffening: may or may not be present
  - Lasts from seconds to less than 60 seconds
- **Pathogenesis:** multifactorial
- **Treatment:** reassurance

Pallid Type

- Onset from the age of 12 to 24 months; gone by 4 to 6 years of age
- Clinical features
  - Child experiencing painful insult or fear
  - May or may not cry, may gasp
  - Loss of consciousness
  - Pallor and diaphoresis
  - Loss of tone
  - Brief tonic-clonic seizure: may or may not be present
- **Mechanism:** vasovagal leading to bradycardia and even asystole
- **Treatment:** reassurance; rarely, atropine may be necessary

Pseudoseizures

- History of epilepsy: may or may not be present
- Movements: semipurposeful and nonstereotypic
- Thrashing, rather than tonic-clonic
- May have pelvic thrusting with opisthotonic posture
- Usually no postictal state
- No injury
- No tongue biting
- Urinary incontinence in 20%
- **Evaluation:** video-electroencephalographic monitoring
- **Treatment:** counseling and reassurance

Suggested Reading

Breningstall GN. Breath-holding spells. *Pediatr Neurol* 1996;14:91–97.

Emery ES. Status epilepticus secondary to breath-holding and pallid syncopal spells. *Neurology* 1990;40:859.

Golden GS. The Alice in Wonderland syndrome in juvenile migraine. *Pediatrics* 1979;63:517–519.

Gordon N. Breath-holding spells. *Dev Med Child Neurol* 1987;29:811–814.

Gummit RJ. Psychogenic seizures. In: Wyllie E, ed. *The treatment of epilepsy: principles and practice.* Philadelphia: Lea & Febiger, 1993:692–696.

Laxdal T, Gomez MR, Reiher J. Cyanotic and pallid syncopal attacks in children (breath-holding spells). *Dev Med Child Neurol* 1969;11:755–763.

Lombroso CT, Lerman P. Breath-holding spells (cyanotic and pallid infantile syncope). *Pediatrics* 1967;39:563–581.

Sallustro C, Atwell F. Body rocking, head-banging, and head-rolling in normal children. *J Pediatr* 1978;93:704–708.

Wyllie E, Friedman D, Luders H, et al. Outcome of psychogenic seizures in children and adolescents compared with adults. *Neurology* 1991;41: 742–744.

Wyllie E, Friedman D, Rothner AD, et al. Psychogenic seizures in children and adolescents: outcome after diagnosis by ictal video and electroencephalographic recording. *Pediatrics* 1990;85:480–484.

Chapter 21

Sleep Disorders

Case

A 2-year-old boy is brought in for evaluation because of frequent episodes of screaming at night. The child appears terrified, and he is inconsolable. The episodes last for 10 to 15 minutes. The child is amnesic for the event.

Diagnosis

Night terrors (*pavor nocturnus*)
He is treated with 2 mg of diazepam at bedtime with complete resolution of symptoms.

DISORDERS OF SLEEP

Narcolepsy

- Onset: 10 to 20 years of age
- Excessive daytime sleepiness
- Cataplexy
- Sleep paralysis
- Hypnagogic hallucinations
- Multiple episodes of sleeping during the day despite adequate sleep at night

Evaluation

- Multiple sleep latency test (rapid eye movement [REM] sleep seen almost immediately)

- Polysomnogram: rule out sleep apnea and nocturnal seizures

Treatment

- Narcolepsy: stimulant drugs
- Cataplexy: tricyclics

Obstructive Sleep Apnea

- Onset: older than 2 years of age
- Diaphragmatic movement independant of absent airflow at the nose and mouth
- May be associated with behavior change and decline in school performance

Etiologies

- Tonsils or adenoids
- Micrognathia
- Obesity
- Medications

Symptoms

- Snoring with episodes of apnea
- Excessive daytime sleepiness
- Frequent arousals
- Hyperactivity
- Failure to thrive
- Morning headaches
- Cardiac failure
- Hypotension

Evaluation

- Polysomnogram: oxygen desaturation independent of diaphragmatic movement
- Electrocardiogram and echocardiogram
- Imaging of the soft tissues of airway

Treatment

- Surgery to remove tonsils and/or adenoids
- Reconstructive surgery
- Tracheostomy
- Bilevel positive airway pressure (BIPAP)

Congenital Central Alveolar Hypoventilation Syndrome ("Ondine's Curse")

- Depression of central ventilatory drive during non-REM sleep
- Increased respiratory response to carbon dioxide
- Episodes of central apnea: common

Evaluation

- Polysomnogram
- Magnetic resonance imaging of the brain
- Magnetic resonance imaging of the upper cervical cord

Treatment

- May require a tracheostomy and/or a ventilator during sleep
- BIPAP

PARASOMNIAS

Pavor Nocturnus (Night Terrors)

Clinical Features

- Onset: 18 months to 5 years of age (peaks in late preschool)
- Occurs in the first third of the night (stage 4, non-REM sleep)
- Child sits up, with sweating, crying out, tachycardia, confusion, crying; he or she is fearful and inconsolable
- Lasts 10 to 20 minutes or longer
- May be associated with sleep walking
- Difficult to arouse
- Amnesia regarding the event

Treatment

- Support
- Diazepam for severe cases
- No long-term complications

Somnambulism (Sleep Walking)

Clinical Features

- Positive family history
- Begins in non-REM sleep, but walking occurs in delta sleep

- Occurs during transition from deeper to lighter stages of sleep
- Begins in delta sleep
- Child wakes, walks or runs—automatisms
- Lasts for several minutes to 1 hour
- Confusional state if awakened
- Difficult to arouse
- Amnesic regarding the event
- Self-limited

Treatment

- Door locks, and gates
- Diazepam at bedtime if severe

Restless Leg Syndrome

Clinical Features

- Need to move the legs because of a disagreeable feeling
- Begins at onset of sleep
- May be associated with attention deficit hyperactivity disorder

Treatment
Carbidopa or dopa agonists are used for the treatment of this condition.

Nocturnal Enuresis

Clinical Features

- May last until early adolescence
- Usually seen between the first and third hours after the onset of sleep during the shift from non-REM to REM sleep
- Tachycardia, tachypnea, and penile erection
- Urination: within 4 minutes of onset
- Difficult to arouse
- Amnesia regarding the event

Evaluation
Exclude the presence of diabetes, seizures, or urinary tract infection.

Treatment

- Imipramine
- Conditioning therapies
- Desmopressin acetate (DDAVP)

Nightmares

- Occur in REM sleep
- Frightening dream
- No amnesia for event

Suggested Reading

Aldrich MS. Narcolepsy. *N Engl J Med* 1990;323:389–394.

Earley C, Allen R. Pergolide and carbidopa/levodopa treatment of restless leg syndrome and periodic leg movements in sleep in a consecutive series of patients. *Sleep* 1996;19:801–810.

Klackenberg G. Incidence of parasomnias in children in a general population. In: Guilleminault C, ed. *Sleep and its disorders in children.* New York: Raven Press, 1987.

Kotagal S, Hartse K, Walsh JK. Characteristics of narcolepsy in preteenaged children. *Pediatrics* 1990;85:205–209.

Mindell JA. Sleep disorders in children [Review]. *Health Psychol* 1993;12: 151–162.

Report of the Therapeutics and Technology Assessment Subcommittee of the American Academy of Neurology. Assessment: techniques associated with the diagnosis and management of sleep disorders. *Neurology* 1992;42:269–275.

Chapter 22

Complications of Antiepileptic Drugs

Case

A 6-year-old girl presented with her second afebrile generalized seizure. She was given phenytoin (20 mg per kg) and was then begun on maintenance therapy. Two weeks later, she developed a maculopapular rash involving her trunk and extremities and a high fever. On examination, she had facial edema and hepatomegaly.

Diagnosis

Phenytoin hypersensitivity syndrome
Phenytoin was immediately discontinued.

Anticonvulsants have a variety of side effects, some of which are idiosyncratic and others that are related to toxic levels of the drug. With all the new antiepileptic drugs (AEDs) available today, identifying the characteristics of the "ideal drug" is useful.

- Ease of administration—especially important in young children
- Oral and parenteral forms (both intravenous and intramuscular)
- Easily monitored
- Wide therapeutic range
- Kinetics unchanged in the therapeutic range
- Acceptable idiosyncratic effects
- Limited drug–drug interactions

- Reasonable cost-to-benefit ratio
- Long half-life

The risk of drug toxicity increases with polypharmacy.

PHENOBARBITAL

Table 22.1 summarizes information about phenobarbital.

Acute Toxicity: Dose Related

- Ataxia and nystagmus
- Lethargy
- Stupor and coma
- Cardiorespiratory depression

Acute Toxicity: Non–Dose Related

- Sedation: adults
- Hyperkinesis: children and the elderly
- Insomnia
- Irritability and change in affect
- Decreased attention span
- Possible adverse effect on cognition

Neonatal Coagulation Defects

- Seen within 24 hours of birth
- Administer vitamin K

TABLE 22.1 Phenobarbital

Ideal Drug	
Ease of administration	+
Give orally and parenterally	+ (p.o., i.m., i.v.)
Easily monitored	+
Wide therapeutic range	+ (15–40 µg/mL)
Does not change kinetics in the therapeutic range	+
Acceptable idiosyncratic effects	±
Limited drug interactions	– (inducer)
Cost-to-benefit reasonable	+
Long half-life	+ (96 h)

Abbreviations: i.m., intramuscular; i.v., intravenous; p.o., oral.

Idiosyncratic Reactions

- Rashes: 1% to 3%
- Stevens-Johnson syndrome

PHENYTOIN (DILANTIN)

Table 22.2 summarizes the effects of Phenytoin (Dilantin).

Acute Toxicity: Dose Related

- Cerebellovestibular (serum level of 20 to 30 μg per mL)
- Higher cortical function (serum level of 40 μg per mL)
- Pyramidal and extrapyramidal
- Seizures increased at serum levels higher than 40 μg per mL
- Coma

Acute Toxicity: Non–Dose Related

- Gingival hyperplasia
- Coarsening of the facial features
- Hirsutism
- Acne
- Neuropathy
- Megaloblastic anemia—prescribe folic acid
- Pseudolymphoma—discontinue phenytoin
- Neonatal coagulation defects
  - Seen within 24 hours of birth
  - Administer vitamin K

TABLE 22.2 Phenytoin (Dilantin)

Ideal Drug	
Ease of administration	+
Give orally and parenterally	+ (p.o., i.v., i.m., fosphenytoin)
Easily monitored	+
Wide therapeutic range	10–20 μg/mL
Does not change kinetics in the therapeutic range	–
Acceptable idiosyncratic effects	–
Limited drug interactions	– (inducer)
Cost-to-benefit reasonable	+
Long half-life	+ (24 h)

Abbreviations: i.m., intramuscular; i.v., intravenous; p.o., oral.

- Decreased thyroxine, normal thyroid-stimulating hormone
  - Competes with thyroxine for binding sites
  - Clinically euthyroid
  - Measure free thyroxine to assess true thyroid level
  - Inhibits glucose-induced insulin release
- Rickets
  - Increased risk of pathologic fractures
  - Decreased calcium
  - Deficiency in 25-hydroxide (OH) cholecalciferol
  - Treatment
    - 4,000 IU vitamin D_2 for 4 months
    - 1,000 IU vitamin D_2 daily maintenance

Idiosyncratic Reactions Affecting the Skin

- Exfoliative dermatitis
- Stevens-Johnson syndrome
- Periarteritis nodosa
- Serum sickness
- Purpura fulminans

Phenytoin Hypersensitivity Reaction

- Begins 1 to 3 weeks after beginning drug
- No relation to drug dose or serum level
- Rash: seen in 100% of patients, maculopapular
- Fever: seen in 50%
- Jaundice: seen in 55%
- Lymphadenopathy: seen in 75%
- Hepatomegaly: seen in 65%
- Splenomegaly: seen in 35%
- Eosinophilia: common
- Increased bilirubin, aspartate aminotransferase, alkaline phosphatase: seen in 70%
- Liver biopsy: hepatitis, fatty infiltration, diffuse cellular necrosis
- Mortality: 18%

Treatment

- Immediate drug withdrawal
- Steroids: may suppress hypersensitivity but increase risk of gastrointestinal hemorrhage

- Intravenous immunoglobulin: promising results in uncontrolled studies

Phenytoin Encephalopathy

- Dementia and behavior disorders
- Psychomotor slowing
- Involuntary movements
- Toxic levels: may or may not be present

CARBAMAZEPINE

Table 22.3 contains additional information about carbamazepine's effects.

Acute Toxicity: Dose Related

- Dizziness
- Diplopia
- Drowsiness
- Headache
- Ataxia
- Arrhythmia (potentially fatal)

Serum levels increase with concomitant use of erythromycin, cimetidine, and verapamil.

Acute Toxicity: Non–Dose Related

- Nausea
- Cardiac conduction blocks

TABLE 22.3 Carbamazepine

Ideal Drug	
Ease of administration	+
Give orally and parenterally	– (p.o.)
Easily monitored	+
Wide therapeutic range	4–12 μg/mL
Does not change kinetics in the therapeutic range	+*
Acceptable idiosyncratic effects	+
Limited drug interactions	– (inducer)
Cost-to-benefit reasonable	±
Long half-life	+ (long-acting preparations)

Abbreviation: p.o., oral.

*Initially induces its own metabolism.

- Blurry vision
- Irritability
- Fluid retention (hyponatremia)
- Urinary frequency (anticholinergic effects on bladder)
- Hematologic
  - Leukopenia: common; maintain absolute neutrophil count (ANC) higher than 1,000 mm^3
  - Thrombocytopenia: rare

Idiosyncratic Reactions

- Aplastic anemia
- Hepatotoxicity
- Hypersensitivity syndrome
  - Rash
  - Eosinophilia
  - Lymphadenopathy
  - Splenomegaly
- Typical AED hypersensitivity syndrome (see phenytoin)

VALPROIC ACID

Table 22.4 has additional information on valproic acid.

Acute Toxicity: Dose Related

- Intention tremor
- Encephalopathy

TABLE 22.4 Valproic Acid

Ideal Drug	
Ease of administration	+
Give orally and parenterally	+ (p.o., i.v.)
Easily monitored	+
Wide therapeutic range	50–100 µg/mL
Does not change kinetics in the therapeutic range	+
Acceptable idiosyncratic effects	–
Limited drug interactions	– (inhibitor)
Cost-to-benefit reasonable	±
Long half-life	± (depends on preparation)

Abbreviations: i.v., intravenous; p.o., oral.

Acute Toxicity: Non–Dose Related

- Nausea
- Weight gain
- Alopecia (nonpermanent)
- Hyperactivity (rare)
- **Hematologic**
  - Thrombocytopenia
    - Occurs with viral infections
    - Prescribe platelets or intravenous immunoglobulin
    - Can resume use when illness is over
  - Increase in bleeding time
  - Easy bruising
- Polycystic ovaries
- Irregular menses

Idiosyncratic Reactions

- Stevens-Johnson syndrome: rare
- Hepatic failure
  - Loss of appetite
  - Nausea and vomiting
  - Edema (periorbital; dependent)
  - Abdominal pain
  - Lethargy
  - Children at greatest risk for hepatic fatality: those who are developmentally delayed, those who have been on polypharmacy; those less than 3 years of age; incidence is 1 per 500
- Pancreatitis

Use in Pregnancy

- Risk for neural tube defects: 1% when taken in first trimester
- Monitor with α-fetoprotein analysis and ultrasonography before week 20
- Give folic acid, 1 mg, to all girls of child-bearing age—decreases risk of neural tube defects in the fetus

NEW AGENTS: LIMITED DRUG–DRUG INTERACTIONS

Felbamate

- Weight loss
- Nausea and vomiting

- Insomnia
- Dizziness
- Aplastic anemia (can be delayed)
- Hepatotoxicity

Felbamate is sufficiently toxic that it should be used only in exceptional circumstances.

Lamotrigine: Idiosyncratic Reactions

- Rash
  - Stevens-Johnson syndrome, toxic epidermal necrolysis—especially in children, the incidence is 1 in 50
  - Increased with use of valproic acid
  - Increased if the drug is advanced too quickly
- Hepatotoxicity

Gabapentin

- Somnolence
- Dizziness
- Lethargy
- Not metabolized in liver
- No drug–drug interactions
- **Idiosyncratic reactions:** none reported as yet

Topiramate

- Speech (word finding) difficulties
- Paresthesias
- Confusion
- Emotional lability
- Weight loss
- **Idiosyncratic reactions**
  - Acute myopia and secondary angle closure glaucoma
  - Renal stones: seen in 1.5% of patients

Vigabitrine

Vigabitrine is not approved by the United States Food and Drug Administration.

- Drowsiness and fatigue
- Dizziness

- Headache
- **Idiosyncratic reactions**
  - Visual field defects
  - Psychosis

Zonisamide

The use of zonisamide is contraindicated in patients with allergies to sulfa-containing drugs.

- Anorexia, nausea
- Headache
- Somnolence
- Difficulty concentrating
- **Idiosyncratic reactions**
  - Stevens-Johnson syndrome
  - Toxic epidermal necrolysis
  - Fulminant hepatic necrosis
  - Agranulocytosis
  - Aplastic anemia
  - Renal stones: seen in 1.9% to 4%; decreased renal function
  - Oligohidrosis and hyperthermia; risk of heat stroke, so monitor for decreased sweating and increased body temperature

Levetiracetam

- Somnolence
- Dizziness
- Nervousness
- Headache
- **Idiosyncratic reactions:** psychotic symptoms

Tiagabine

- Abdominal pain and nausea
- Dizziness
- Somnolence
- Tremor
- Irritability
- Difficulty with concentration
- **Idiosyncratic reactions:** serious rash

Oxcarbazepine

- Headache
- Diplopia
- Ataxia
- Abnormal vision
- Nausea and vomiting
- Tremor
- Somnolence
- **Idiosyncratic reactions**
  - Hyponatremia
  - Stevens-Johnson syndrome
  - Angioedema
  - Hepatotoxicity
  - Leukopenia

TERATOGENICITY

Incidence

- Epileptic mothers with AED: 6%
- Epileptic mothers without AED: 4.2%
- Nonepileptic mothers: 2%

Features of the Fetal Anticonvulsant Syndrome

- Limb abnormalities
  - Digital hypoplasia of the terminal phalanges
  - Small or absent nails of the fingers and toes
- Craniofacial abnormalities
  - Short nose and low nasal bridge
  - Hypertelorism
  - Epicanthal folds
  - Ptosis
  - Strabismus
  - Low-set ears
  - Wide mouth, prominent lips
  - Cleft palate
- Growth and development abnormalities
  - Microcephaly
  - Trigonocephaly
  - Mental deficiency
  - Short stature

Suggested Reading

American Academy of Pediatrics, Committee on Drugs. Behavioral and cognitive effects of anticonvulsant therapy. *Pediatrics* 1995;76:538–540.

Devinsky O, Cramer J. Safety and efficacy of standard and new antiepileptic drugs. *Neurology* 2000;55:S5–S10.

Glauser TA. Idiosyncratic reactions: new methods of identifying high-risk patients. *Epilepsia* 2000;41:S16–S29.

Haruda F. Phenytoin hypersensitivity: 38 cases. *Neurology* 1979;29:1480–1485.

Holmes LB. Teratogenic effects of anticonvulsant drugs. *Pediatrics* 1988;112: 579–581.

Isojärvi JI, Laatikainen TJ, Pakarinen AJ, et al. Polycystic ovaries and hyperandrogenism in women taking valproate for epilepsy. *N Engl J Med* 1993;329:1383–1388.

Meador KJ, Gilliam FG, Kanner AM, et al. Cognitive and behavioral effects of antiepileptic drugs. *Epilepsy Behav* 2001;2:SS1–SS17.

Meador KJ, Loring DW, Hu K, et al. Comparative cognitive effects of anticonvulsants. *Neurology* 1990;40:391–394.

Mitchell AA, Lacouture PG, Sheehan JE, et al. Adverse drug reactions in children leading to hospital admission. *Pediatrics* 1988;82:24–29.

Moss D, Rudis M, Henderson SO. Cross-sensitivity and the anticonvulsant hypersensitivity syndrome. *Pharmacol Emerg Med* 1999;17:503–506.

Pellock JM. Efficacy and adverse effects of antiepileptic drugs. *Pediatr Clin North Am* 1989;36:435–447.

Pellock JM, Watemberg N. New antiepileptic drugs in children: present and future. *Semin Pediatr Neurol* 1997;4:9–18.

Pollack MA, Burk PG, Nathanson G. Mucocutaneous eruptions due to antiepileptic drug therapy in children. *Ann Neurol* 1979;5:262–267.

Powers NG, Carson SH. Idiosyncratic reactions to phenytoin. *Clin Pediatr* 1987;26:120–124.

Prosser TR, Lander RD. Phenytoin-induced hypersensitivity reactions. *Clin Pharmacol* 1987;6:728–734.

Roujeau JC, Stern RS. Severe adverse cutaneous reactions to drugs. *N Engl J Med* 1994;331:1272–1286.

Scheuerman O, Moses YN, Rachmel A, et al. Successful treatment of antiepileptic drug hypersensitivity syndrome with intravenous immune globulin. *Pediatrics* 2001;107:1–2.

White HS. Comparative anticonvulsant and mechanistic profile of the established and newer antiepileptic drugs. *Epilepsia* 1999;40:S2–S10.

Chapter 23

Genetics

Case

A 2-year-old boy presents with a history of developmental delay. He has large testicles, repetitive speech, and attention deficit disorder. He has a brother with the same problem and a sister who is normal with some suggested learning disabilities. DNA-based molecular analysis is obtained; it reveals a CGG triplicate repeat.

Diagnosis

Fragile X syndrome (see Chapter 13)

Increasingly, as a result of the completion of the genomic project, genetic syndromes of the nervous system are being identified and codified. Mendelian inheritance suggests that information in the nucleus is encoded by DNA and then transcripted from DNA to RNA. Messenger RNA consists of transcripts of DNA that encode polypeptides. The process of polypeptide synthesis that takes place in the cytosome is called translation. The human nuclear genome consists of approximately 30,000 genes, although some have suggested that the number of genes may be as high as 70,000. Repeat sequences are thought to occupy from 6% to 10% of the genome.

The human genome consists of 22 matched chromosomes or 44 autosomal chromosomes and two sex chromosomes—XY or XX—depending on the gender of the individual. Various staining techniques are used to identify the individual chromosomes. A nomenclature for classifying chromosomes was developed in 1995; it uses a method that segregates genes into regions and subregions. The letter "p" is used to identify the short arm, whereas "q" is used to denote the long arm of the chromosome. Mutations represent permanent changes in the DNA. Mutations may be replication errors, deletions, substitutions, duplications, or insertions. To have a normal number of chromosomes, the individual must have the correct number of chromosomes, both haploid and diploid. Aneuploidy is any number that derives from a multiple of the haploid number. Although most monosomies and trisomies are lethal, a few produce clinical syndromes, such as Prader-Willi, 45XO, and trisomy 21. Triploidy and even tetraploidy (i.e., three or four times the haploid number) are extraordinarily rare. Southern blotting analysis is the procedure of hybridizing single-stranded DNA and then exposing it to x-ray film to determine where the hybridized probe has been labeled.

The most common patterns of inheritance are as follows:

- **Autosomal dominant**
  - Offspring have a 50% chance of inheriting the defect, if one parent is heterozygous and the other is normal.
  - Offspring of unaffected individuals are not affected.
  - The defect may be transferred from either parent.
  - Spontaneous mutations may occur.
- **Autosomal recessive**
  - If both parents are heterozygous, then the following will be true of the offspring:
    - Chance of being normal is 25%.
    - Chance of expressing the trait is 25%.
    - Chance of being a carrier of the trait is 50%.
  - If only one parent is heterozygous and the other is homozygous dominant, then the following will be true of the offspring:
    - Fifty percent will be normal.
    - Fifty percent will be carriers.
- **X-linked inheritance**
  - Incidence is much higher in males but not inevitable.
  - The gene is transmitted through an affected female.
  - With a carrier mother, males have a 50% chance of contracting the disease; 50% of the females will be carriers.
  - Most X-linked illnesses are recessive. X-linked dominant implies that both males and females are affected.
  - X-linked dominant disease is seen in females, and it suggests lethality in the male (e.g., ornithine transcarbamylase (OTC) deficiency).

- ◆ Lionization refers to the inactivation of a normal X chromosome that results from the expression of the abnormal active X chromosome.

MITOCHONDRIAL DISEASE

Mitochondria are the cellular organelles that are intimately involved in intermediate metabolism. All mitochondrial DNA is derived from the mother's ovum. This alone accounts for the observation that disease of the mitochondrion is derived exclusively from the mother. Inheritance is largely nonmendelian, and it, for the most part, is expressed randomly. Phenotype is determined by the relative proportion of wild to mutated genomes. However, not all disease of the mitochondrion is inherited in a matrilineal fashion. Most mitochondrial diseases that affect the Krebs cycle and the diseases of fatty acid oxidation are inherited in a mendelian fashion; that is, they are determined by nuclear genetics and not mitochondrial genetics.

Examples of Matrilineal Inheritance (Mitochondrial DNA)

- Kearns-Sayre syndrome
- Myoclonic epilepsy with ragged red fibers (MERRF)
- Mitochondrial encephalomyelopathy with lactic acidosis and strokelike episodes (MELAS)
- Leber optic atrophy

Examples of Nuclear Inheritance

- Pyruvate dehydrogenase deficiency
- Pyruvate carboxylase deficiency
- Respiratory chain abnormalities (e.g., Leigh syndrome)
- β-Oxidation defects

Clues to Diagnosis of Mitochondrial Disease: Clinical and Laboratory Features

- Acidosis
  - ◆ Increased lactate to pyruvate ratio
  - ◆ Increased lactate, normal pyruvate
  - ◆ Progressive weakness
  - ◆ Ragged red fibers on muscle biopsy
  - ◆ Cognitive loss
  - ◆ Microcephaly
  - ◆ Optic atrophy

- Neuroimaging
  - Ventricular dilatation
  - Increase in T2-weighted signals in the caudate, putamen, and globus pallidus
  - Changes in the basal ganglia
  - Myelin loss
  - Increase in T2-weighted signals in the white matter
  - Cerebral infarct pattern, usually in the posterior cerebral hemispheres
- Gross pathology
  - Myelin loss
  - Proliferation of microvessels
  - Destruction of the brainstem, thalamus, basal ganglia, and cerebellum; encephalomalacia
  - Spongy encephalopathy
  - Microcephaly
  - Malformations
- Destructive lesion of the brain
  - Magnetic resonance imaging hyperintensities in the basal ganglia
  - Stroke-like lesions
  - Demyelination
  - Encephalomalacia

TRINUCLEOTIDE REPEATS

Trinucleotide repeats (Table 23.1) are diseases associated with an increased number of oligonucleotides. For the most part,

TABLE 23.1 Diseases of Trinucleotide Repeats

	Repeat	Chromosome
DRPLA	CAG	12p
Fragile X syndrome	CGG	Xq
Friedreich ataxia	GAA	9q
Huntington disease	CAG	4p
Myotonic dystrophy type 1	CTG	19q
Myotonic dystrophy type 2	CCTG	3q
Spinocerebellar ataxia type 1	CAG	6p
Spinocerebellar ataxia type 2	CAG	12q
Spinocerebellar ataxia type 3	CAG	14q
Spinocerebellar ataxia type 6	CAG	19p
Spinocerebellar ataxia type 7	CAG	3p

Abbreviation: DRPLA, dentatorubral-pallidoluysian atrophy.

TABLE 23.2 Diseases of Lysosomes

Disease	Enzyme Defect	Substance Stored	Gene Location
Glycogenosis Disorders			
Pompe disease	Acid-α1,4-glucosidase	Glycogen α-1, 4-linked oligosaccharides	17
Glycolipidosis Disorders			
G_{M1} Gangliosidosis	β-Galactosidase	G_{M1} ganglioside	3
Tay-Sachs disease	β-Hexosaminidase A	G_{M2} ganglioside	15
G_{M2} gangliosidosis, AB variant	G_{M2} activator protein	G_{M2} ganglioside	5
Sandhoff disease	β-Hexosaminidase A and B	G_{M2} ganglioside	5
Fabry disease	α-Galactosidase A	Globosides	X
Gaucher disease	Glucocerebrosidase	Glucosylceramide	1
Metachromatic leukodystrophy	Arylsulfatase A	Sulphatides	22
Krabbe disease	Galactosylceramidase	Galactocerebroside	14
Niemann-Pick, types A and B	Sphingomyelinase	Sphingomyelin	
Niemann-Pick, type C	Cholesterol esterification defect	Sphingomyelin	18
Niemann-Pick, type D	Unknown	Sphingomyelin	18
Farber disease	Acid ceramidase	Ceramide	18
Wolman disease (mucopolysaccharidosis)	Acid lipase	Cholesteryl esters	?
Hurler syndrome (MPS IH)	α-L-Iduronidase	Heparan and dermatan sulfates	10
Scheie syndrome (MPS IS)	α-L-Iduronidase	Heparan and dermatan sulfates	4
Hurler-Scheie (MPS I H/S)	α-L-Iduronidase	Heparan and dermatan sulfates	4
Hunter syndrome (MPS II)	Iduronate sulfatase	Heparan and dermatan sulfates	4
Sanfilippo A (MPS III A)	Heparan *N*-sulfatase	Heparan sulfate	X
			17

(Continued)

TABLE 23.2 (Continued)

Disease	Enzyme Defect	Substance Stored	Gene Location
Sanfilippo B (MPS III B)	α-*N*-acetylglucosaminidase	Heparan sulfate	17
Sanfilippo C (MPS III C)	Acetyl-CoA-glucosaminide acetyltransferase	Heparan sulfate	14
Sanfilippo D (MPS III D)	*N*-acetylglucosamine-6-sulfatase	Heparan sulfate	12
Morquio A (MPS IV A)	Galactosamine-6-sulfatase	Keratan	16
Morquio B (MPS IV B)	β-Galactosidase	Keratan sulfate	3
Maroteaux-Lamy (MPS VI)	Arylsulfatase β	Dermatan sulfate	5
Sly syndrome	β-Glucuronidase	?	7
Oligosaccharide/Glycoprotein Disorders			
α-Mannosidosis	α-Mannosidase	Mannose/oligosaccharides	19
β-Mannosidosis	β-Mannosidase	Mannose/oligosaccharides	4
Fucosidosis	α-L-Fucosidase	Fucosyl oligosaccharides	1
Asparylglucosaminuria	*N*-Aspartyl-β-glucosaminidase	Asparylglucosamine, Asparagines	4
Sialidosis (mucolipidosis I)	α-Neuraminidase	Sialyloligosaccharides	20
Galactosialidosis (Goldberg syndrome)	Lysosomal protective protein deficiency	Sialyloligosaccharides	20
Schindler disease	α-*N*-Acetyl galactosaminidase	?	22

Lysosomal Enzyme Transport Disorders			
Mucolipidosis II (I-cell disease)	*N*-Acetylglucosamine-1-phosphotransferase	Heparan sulfate	4
Mucolipidosis III (Pseudo-Hurler polydystrophy)	Same as mucolipidosis II		4
Lysosomal Membrane Transport Disorders			
Cystinosis	Cystine transport protein	Free cystine	17
Salla disease	Sialic acid transport protein	Free sialic acid and glucuronic acid	6
Infantile sialic acid storage disease	Sialic acid transport protein	Free sialic acid and glucuronic acid	6
Other			
Batten disease (juvenile neuronal ceroid lipofuscinosis)	Unknown	Lipofuscins	16
Infantile neuronal ceroid lipofuscinosis	Palmitoyl-protein thioesterase	Lipofuscins	1
Mucolipidosis IV	Unknown	Gangliosides and hyaluronic acid	?
Prosaposin	Saposins A, B, C, or D	—	10

Abbreviation: MPS, mucopolysaccharidosis.

Modified from *Lysosomal storage diseases: a family sourcebook reference chart.* Available at: http://mcrcr2.med.nyu.edu/murphp01/lysosome/lysosome.htm and http://www.genetests.org. Accessed September 29, 1999, with permission.

the severity of the disease type relates directly to the number of repeats. These diseases are associated with the phenomenon of anticipatory inheritance. This suggests that an affected individual's progeny are apt to be more severely infected and to have evidence of more repeats than are seen in the parent. At least 10 known diseases are associated with trinucleotide repeats. Myotonic dystrophy, spinocerebellar degenerations, and fragile X are of major pediatric interest (see Chapter 9).

DISEASES OF LYSOSOMES

Lysosomes are subcellular vesicles that contain enzymes responsible for the degradation of catabolic products. Defects and the absence of enzymatic processes characterize lysosomal disease (Table 23.2). These abnormalities are, for the most part, recessive.

Suggested Reading

Baraitser M. *The genetics of neurologic disorders.* Oxford: Oxford University Press, 1999.

Chance PF, Fishbeck KH. Molecular genetics of Charcot-Marie-Tooth disease and related neuropathies. *Hum Mol Genet* 1994;3 Spec. No.:1503–1507.

Dobyns WB. Introduction to genetics. In: Swaiman KF, Ashwal S, eds. *Pediatric neurology: principles and practice,* 3rd ed. St. Louis: Mosby, 1999.

Harding AE, Rosenberg RN. A neurologic gene map. In: Rosenberg RN, Prusiner SB, DiMauro S, Barchi RL, eds. *The molecular and genetic basis of neurological disease,* 2nd ed. Boston: Butterworth-Heinemann, 1997:23–28.

McKusick VA. *Mendelian inheritance in man: a catalog of human genes and genetic disorders,* 11th ed. Baltimore: Johns Hopkins University Press, 1994.

Rimoin DL, Connor JM, Pyeritz RE, eds. *Emery and Rimoin's principles and practice of medical genetics,* 3rd ed. New York: Churchill Livingston, 1997.

Thompson MW, McInnes RR, Willard HF. *Genetics of medicine,* 5th ed. Philadelphia: WB Saunders, 1991.

Chapter 24

Headaches

Case

A 7-year-old boy presents with headaches that are diffuse and throbbing. No aura is present. He is photophobic and sonophobic during the headaches. He also becomes nauseated with the headaches and then vomits. Going to sleep relieves them. They occur one to two times per month. His father also had headaches as a child. The child's neurologic examination is normal.

Diagnosis

Juvenile migraine

Headaches are a common complaint in children, yet the etiologies are diverse, ranging in severity from mass lesions to anxiety-related causes. A careful analysis of the child's symptoms and physical examination will, in most cases, lead to the correct diagnosis.

SYMPTOMS

1. **Tempo and progression**
   - *Mass lesion:* gradual increase in headache over time. In very young children with mass lesions, the tempo and/or progression may have a biphasic character. The child may complain of headaches for several weeks that then abate as

sutural diastasis occurs, only to resurface when the pressure becomes excessive.

- *Migraine:* headache that has a crescendo and decrescendo pattern, separated by symptom-free intervals.
- *Tension:* headaches that occur daily with only mild fluctuation in intensity, usually reflecting underlying tension and stress.

2. **Location.** The location of the headache is important, even though headaches in general reflect referred pain (anterior and middle cranial fossa pain is referred to the ophthalmic division of cranial nerve V and posterior fossa pain is referred to cranial nerves IX and X, C1 and 2). Localization is important if the pain is always in the same region.
3. **Time of day.** Questioning the child as to what time of day the headaches occur is important—whether they occur first thing in the morning or in the afternoon or if they wake the child from sleep. Differentiating the child who cannot get to sleep because of anxiety versus the child who is sound asleep and who then wakes with severe headache is particularly important.
4. **Headaches that increase with Valsalva maneuvers.** If the headache increases with Valsalva maneuvers (i.e., with coughing, sneezing, or during a bowel movement), increased intracranial pressure should be excluded.
5. **Quality of pain.** The quality of pain is often difficult to determine in a very young child who may have difficulty describing the pain. The adolescent can typically describe the throbbing, pulsatile feeling of a migraine versus the pressure sensation of a tension headache.
6. **Vomiting.** Vomiting is a characteristic feature of both increased intracranial pressure and migraine, but it is unusual in tension headaches.
7. **Neck stiffness.** If the child develops neck stiffness and/or pain with a severe headache, subarachnoid hemorrhage or meningitis should be excluded. In addition, incipient cerebellar herniation is associated with neck pain due to irritation of the cervical roots.
8. **Associated visual or motor symptoms.** Asking whether associated visual or motor symptoms are present either preceding, occurring concurrently with, or beginning after the headache is particularly important.

Warning Symptoms

Patients with the following complaints deserve a complete neurologic evaluation to exclude a mass lesion:

- Recurrent morning headaches—also consider hypercarbia associated with sleep apnea
- Headaches that wake the child from sleep
- Persistently focal headaches
- Headaches that increase with Valsalva maneuvers
- Headaches that have changed in quality, frequency, or pattern over time
- Headaches associated with vomiting
- Headaches associated with behavioral change
- Headaches associated with change in school performance

Physical Examination

A detailed general and neurologic examination is necessary to arrive at a specific diagnosis. Parts of the neurologic exam of particular importance are as follows:

- *Head circumference.* A change in percentile is cause for more concern than is a head circumference that is in the 90th percentile. The change in percentile may suggest increased intracranial pressure causing sutural diastasis in the young child with subsequent growth of the head.
- *Visual and extraocular movement abnormalities*
  - Cranial nerve II
    - Papilledema
    - Optic atrophy (secondary to chronic increased intracranial pressure)
    - Visual acuity (normal with papilledema but abnormal with optic atrophy)
    - Visual fields
  - Cranial nerve IV. The child who presents with a head tilt merits concern because children may tilt their heads either because of a fourth nerve palsy or because the cerebellar tonsils are irritating the cervical roots, which suggests incipient tonsillar herniation.
  - Cranial nerve VI. The child who does not fill the outer canthus on lateral gaze may have a sixth nerve palsy. Although young children will only rarely complain of double vision,

they tend to close one eye or to turn their heads to obscure the double image.
  - Failure of upward gaze. The child who cannot look directly upward may have a pineal region tumor that is compressing the quadrigeminal plate.
- *Cutaneous lesions.* The child who presents with headache who also has ash-leaf spots, adenoma sebaceum, shagreen patches, periungual fibromas, and/or phakomas in the eye may have tuberous sclerosis. In this case, the child's headaches may reflect obstruction at the level of the foramen of Monro that is secondary to a giant cell astrocytoma. Moreover, the child who presents with café-au-lait spots or axillary or inguinal freckling likely has neurofibromatosis, which is frequently associated with intracranial mass lesions.
- *Focal motor signs, ataxia, or reflex asymmetries.* These merit a complete investigation. Most headaches are not associated with mass lesions. In children with headache for at least 8 weeks, one study found that 85% of patients had clear-cut ocular signs and that, by 6 months, all of the children had evidence of structural disease on neurologic examination. In another study, 98% of children with supratentorial tumors and headaches had at least one neurologic abnormality on examination, as did 99% of children with intratentorial tumors and headaches. **Although the diagnosis of a mass lesion is usually straightforward, a vascular malformation can closely mimic the symptoms of migraine in the presence of a normal neurologic examination.**

MIGRAINE HEADACHES

Migraine is a common cause of headaches in children. Migraines can occur at any age, and they have been reported in the first 2 years of life. The peak incidence is between 6 and 10 years of age. They occur more commonly in boys than in girls. A previous diagnosis of motion sickness, sea sickness, or cyclic vomiting is commonly elicited.

Definition

According to Prensky, recurrent headaches separated by symptom-free intervals and any *three* of the following symptoms:

- Abdominal pain
- Nausea and vomiting
- Hemicrania
- A throbbing, pulsatile quality to the pain
- Complete relief after a period of rest
- An aura: visual, sensory, or motor
- A family history of migraine

Differences Between Juvenile and Adult Migraine

- Juvenile migraine is more common in boys than in girls, whereas adult migraine is more common in women than in men.
- Children are more likely to have migraine without aura, whereas adults are more likely to have migraine with aura.
- Nausea and vomiting are common in both adults and children, although abdominal pain is more common in children.
- Children tend to have diffuse headaches, whereas adults more often have hemicrania.
- A history of seizures is reported in up to 10% of children with migraine, but this association is rare in adults.

Classification

- Migraine with aura
- Migraine without aura
- Complicated migraine
- Migraine variants

Migraine with Aura

- Visual loss, scotomata, and hemianopsia (aura): precede the headache
- Unilateral throbbing pain over the eye, temple, and forehead
- Nausea and vomiting
- Anorexia
- Photophobia and sonophobia
- Need for sleep
- Recovery

Migraine Without Aura

No aura is present, and the headaches are bifrontal. The remainder of the headache syndrome is the same.

Complicated Migraine

- *Hemiplegic migraine:* associated with transient focal neurologic deficits lasting hours to days. It has an autosomal dominant inheritance in some families, which has been linked to chromosome 19.
- *Basilar artery migraine:* occurs in 3% to 19% of patients with juvenile migraine; most common in adolescence. The signs and symptoms reflect vasoconstriction in the posterior circulation; they are characterized by dizziness, vertigo, visual disturbances, ataxia, ocular motor dysfunction, visual field abnormalities, and even syncope. The symptoms can last from minutes to hours, and they are typically followed by an occipital headache.
- *Ophthalmoplegic migraine:* often associated with a painful ophthalmoparesis. Patients may complain of blurred vision or diplopia. The third nerve is typically involved, leading to ptosis, limited adduction of eye movements, and an occasional dilated pupil. The eye signs appear *after* the onset of the headache, rather than as an aura, and may persist for 2 weeks after the conclusion of the headache. Occasionally, ophthalmoplegic migraine involves the sixth or, less commonly, the fourth nerve.
- *Acute confusional migraine:* typically occurs in boys; it is associated with agitation, restlessness, disorientation, and occasionally a combative state that usually resolves within 12 hours. Headache and vomiting may precede the confusional state, but, in some, the headache occurs afterward. Episodes may be recurrent in about 25% of patients. At times, the syndrome may be precipitated by minor head trauma.
- *Alice in Wonderland syndrome:* most commonly seen in children; distortion of visual images, such as micropsia, macropsia, and metamorphopsia, is described. Visual symptoms may occur before the headache or at the onset, and, in some cases, headache is not a prominent component of the episode.
- *Cluster headache*
  - Seen in boys far more often than in girls
  - Seen in those older than 10 years of age
  - Clusters of headaches that recur over weeks or months, then resolution for 1 to 2 years
  - Bursts of headache for 30 to 90 minutes

- Always unilateral: begins around the eye and then spreads
- Injected conjunctiva, nasal stuffiness, Horner syndrome, tearing, ipsilateral to the headache
- Intense pain
- Patient walks around rather than lying down as in migraine
- **Treatment**
  - Methysergide maleate
  - Corticosteroids
  - Tryptans

- *Chronic paroxysmal hemicrania*
  - Unilateral
  - Ipsilateral autonomic features
  - Throbbing
  - Frontal and retroorbital
  - Duration is shorter than the cluster headache, but occurs more frequently
  - **Treatment:** indomethacin, acetazolamide
- *Hemicrania continua*
  - Continuous
  - Unilateral
  - Moderate intensity
  - Lasts weeks to months with no remissions
  - **Treatment:** indomethacin

Migraine Variants

- *Benign paroxysmal vertigo:* typically occurs in children between 2 and 6 years of age. A sudden onset of unsteadiness, vertigo, pallor, and nystagmus occurs. Episodes are brief, lasting only a few minutes, and they may or may not be followed by sleep. Vomiting may also occur. Headaches do not accompany the vertigo. Many of these children will go on to develop typical migraine when they grow up.
- *Cyclic vomiting:* begins in early childhood. This is a syndrome of repeated stereotyped episodes of pernicious vomiting that do not stop unless oral intake is discontinued. These children often become typical migraineurs in later life.
- *Paroxysmal torticollis:* syndrome occurring in young children in which recurrent episodes of head tilt are associated with headache, nausea, and vomiting. Symptoms may last from hours to days.

Neurodiagnostic Evaluation

In the child with a normal neurologic examination whose history does not raise any of the "red flags" discussed earlier in this chapter and headaches that have lasted for more than 6 months, routine neuroimaging is *not* indicated. Per the American Academy of Neurology Quality Standards Subcommittee, electroencephalograms are not indicated. If an image is obtained, it should be either a computed tomography with contrast or a magnetic resonance image if the clinician suspects a mass in the midline or posterior fossa or the temporal lobes.

Factors Triggering or Exacerbating Migraines

- Foods
  - Chocolate
  - Cheese
  - Foods containing nitrites (processed meats)
  - Nitrates
  - Monosodium glutamate
  - Red wine
- Caffeine withdrawal
- Drugs
  - Vasodilating drugs
  - Birth control pills: should be avoided as these cause migraines that are hard to control and may be associated with an increased risk of stroke
- Hormonal changes
  - Migraines typically increase the week before menses and during ovulation.
  - These should be treated with acetazolamide, 250 mg twice daily, the week before and the week of menses.
- Stress: migraine headaches may increase both during stressful periods and when the high stress peak is over.

Treatment of Migraine

Children

Placing the child in a quiet room, offering analgesics, and letting the child sleep is usually sufficient to resolve the headache.

Adolescents

- Acetaminophen, ibuprofen
- Butabarbital, caffeine, and acetaminophen (may cause rebound headaches)

- 5-Hydroxytryptamine agonists: not approved for children, studies show limited efficacy
- Avoid narcotics

Prophylaxis

The generally accepted approach is to withhold prophylaxis in children with migraine unless they have more than one or two severe attacks a month. Although very limited double-blind efficacy studies have been conducted in children, the following are regimens that the authors have used successfully:

- Cyproheptadine: 2 to 4 mg twice a day. Side effects include weight gain and lethargy. The agent can generally be discontinued after 3 to 4 months.
- Propranolol: 2 to 4 mg per kg per day, up to a maximum of 120 to 240 mg per day. Has been effective in adults; in children, the results have been contradictory.
- Amitriptyline: particularly effective in adults and adolescents who have a combination of migraine and tension headaches; not well studied in children.
- Anticonvulsants: valproic acid, carbamazepine, gabapentin, and topiramate have become increasingly used in the treatment of childhood migraine.
- Behavioral approaches: both relaxation techniques and self-hypnosis have been helpful in some children with migraine and tension headaches.

TENSION HEADACHES

- Constant, aching, tightness (band around head)
- Back of head and neck
- No nausea, vomiting, photophobia, audiophobia
- Bilateral and diffuse
- Dull and aching
- **Treatment**
  - Amitriptyline
  - Relaxation exercises
  - Counseling

Suggested Reading

American Academy of Neurology. Practice parameter: the utility of neuroimaging in the evaluation of headache in patients with normal neurologic examinations (summary statement). Report of the Quality

Standards Subcommittee of the American Academy of Neurology. *Neurology* 1994;44:1353–1354.

Barlow CR. *Headaches and migraine in childhood.* Philadelphia: JB Lippincott, 1984.

Deonna T, Martin D. Benign paroxysmal torticollis in infancy. *Arch Dis Child* 1981;56:956–959.

Hamalainen ML, Hoppu K, Santavuori P. Sumatriptan for migraine attacks in children: a randomized placebo-controlled study. *Neurology* 1997;48:1100–1103.

Keonigsberger M, Chutorian AM, Gold AP, et al. Benign paroxysmal vertigo of childhood. *Neurology* 1970;20:1108–1113.

Lanzi G, Balottin U, Fazzi E, et al. Benign paroxysmal vertigo of childhood: a long-term follow-up. *Cephalalgia* 1994;14:458–460.

Lapkin M, Golden G. Basilar artery migraine: a review of 30 cases. *Am J Dis Child* 1978;132:278–281.

Lewis DW, Ashwal S, Dahl G, et al. Practice parameter: evaluation of children and adolescents with recurrent headaches. *Neurology* 2002;59:490–498.

Prensky AL. Migraine and migrainous variants in pediatric patients. *Pediatr Clin North Am* 1976;23:461–471.

Rothner AD. Headaches in children and adolescents. *Psychiatr Clin North Am* 1999;8:727–745.

Silbersten SD, Lipton RB. Overview of diagnosis and treatment of migraine. *Neurology* 1994;44:6–16.

Vijayan N. Ophthalmoplegic migraine: ischemic or compressive neuropathy. *Headache* 1980;20:300–304.

Chapter 25

Large Heads, Small Heads

Case

A 5-year-old boy is referred to the office because of a head circumference that is more than the 95th percentile for age. His neurologic examination is normal. He is doing well in school. His neuroimaging is unremarkable. Measurement of the mother's head size reveals a head circumference of 60 cm.

Diagnosis

Familial macrocephaly of no neurologic consequence

Head circumference measurement is one of the most important, if not the most significant, parts of the pediatric neurologic examination. The size of the human brain and, hence indirectly, the head circumference, stays within a remarkably narrow range for all individuals, regardless of the height or weight of the individual. The head circumference of males at birth and throughout life is a bit larger than that of the female. An individual's head circumference reaches approximately 80% of its adult size at 1 year of age. A rule of thumb suggests that the head grows 2 cm a month for the first 3 months, 1 cm a month for the next 3 months, and 0.5 cm per month for the next 6 months (12 cm in the first year of life). Any child whose head circumference measures two standard deviations above or below the mean merits further investigation. Investigation should also be undertaken if head growth either accelerates or falls off the growth chart. If the plot of the head circumference crosses two isobars over several months, investigation is also warranted (see Chapter 1).

ASYMMETRICAL SHAPE

- Rule out synostosis—head growth occurs perpendicular to the line of closure. Therefore, sagittal synostosis is associated with scaphocephaly. Unilateral lambdoid and coronal synostosis is associated with plagiocephaly. Closure of the metopic suture is associated with trigonocephaly. Bilateral coronal synostosis is associated with brachycephaly.
- Porencephaly may cause parietal bulging.
- Dandy-Walker malformations are associated with a large posterior fossa and upward displacement of the external occipital protuberance, the torcular and the transverse sinuses, and the tentorium.
- Brachycephaly and bifrontal prominence are associated with a small posterior fossa, such as is seen in obstructive hydrocephalus secondary to aqueductal stenosis.
- A small head, small maxilla, and exophthalmus suggest Crouzon disease or global synostosis.
- Splitting of the sutures with bulging fontanelle suggests increased intracranial pressure.
- The persistence of wide-open fontanelles may be associated with hypophosphatasia, hypothyroidism, or trisomy 21.
- A gradual decline in head growth in females suggests Rett syndrome.

MACROCEPHALY

Definition

Macrocephaly is defined as more than two standard deviations above the mean. Because fusion of cranial sutures may not be completed until 10 years of age, papilledema may not result in the presence of increased intracranial pressure. This is true because the head expands to accommodate the increased pressure as a result of diastasis of the cranial sutures.

Etiologies

Hydrocephalus

- Communicating hydrocephalus should be differentiated from noncommunicating hydrocephalus. Communicating hydrocephalus is defined as an open ventricular system with failure of the cerebrospinal fluid to be absorbed by passive pressure diffusion through the arachnoid villi into the sagittal sinus. This most commonly results from basilar arachnoiditis secondary to either previous bleeding or infection.
- Noncommunicating hydrocephalus implies a block in the ventricular outflow system. This commonly occurs at the narrowest point of the ventricular system (i.e., the aqueduct cerebri). Technically, noncommunicating obstructive hydrocephalus is defined as a failure of communication between the ventricular outflow tract and the spinal subarachnoid space.
- Other points of cerebrospinal fluid outflow obstruction are at the foramen of Monro and the fourth ventricle (Fig. 25.1).

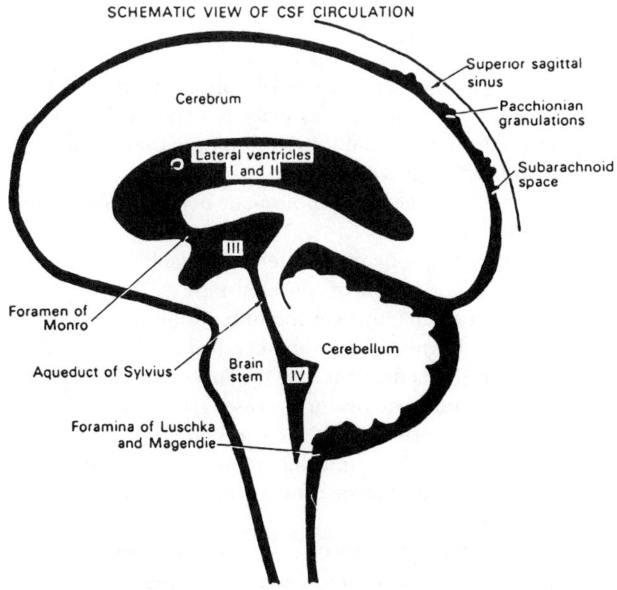

FIGURE 25.1. Cerebrospinal fluid dynamics.

Subdural Hematoma

In infants, look for retinal hemorrhages that are associated with decreased hemoglobulin or hematocrit. In the child older than 6 months of age, the tamponade effect of intracranial bleeding prevents significant loss of blood. Thus, in the child with a low hematocrit, an alternative site of bleeding should be sought. Consider shaken baby syndrome secondary to child abuse in any child with a bulging fontanelle retinal hemorrhages, or other signs of intracranial bleeding.

Subdural Effusions

These are commonly identified in the first several years of life in otherwise healthy children. They usually occur secondary to insignificant trauma from childbirth. More serious causes of subdural effusions are dehydration, trauma, leukemia, and meningitis.

Familial Macrocephaly

The head circumference of the parents should be measured.

Arnold-Chiari Malformation

- *Type I:* the medulla and cerebellar tonsils are displaced caudally, resulting in downward displacement of the fourth ventricle, creating the potential for developing either communicating or obstructive hydrocephalus.
  - Patients usually become symptomatic in early adolescence or early adulthood.
  - Presenting symptoms are either a headache, increased reflexes, or a sudden loss of consciousness.
- *Type II:* the medulla and cerebellum, along with the fourth ventricle, are herniated into the cervical canal. The cervical roots are compressed and course upward to exit from their respective foramina. The posterior fossa is small, and associated developmental anomalies of the cerebellum may be present. Syringomyelia and hydromyelia are associated findings, as is hydrocephalus. Lumbar or thoracic meningomyelocele is invariably present.
- *Type III:* this type is a more severe developmental anomaly than type II, with associated cervical meningomyeloceles or encephalocele.

Holoprosencephaly

- This developmental defect must be differentiated from congenital hydrocephalus.
- It may be lobar or semilobar.
- Intellect is always abnormal, and it can be moderately to severely impaired.

Neoplasms

Tumors may cause an enlarged head as a result of an increased mass or increased volume. Volume increase results from hydrocephalus secondary to the obstruction of cerebrospinal fluid outflow at the foramen of Monro, the aqueduct cerebri, or the fourth ventricle. Increased mass results from growth of tumor anywhere in the brain (see Chapter 26).

Storage Disease

This consists of an increase in brain substance secondary to the accumulation of abnormal brain metabolites (e.g., Alexander and Canavan disease) (see Chapter 13).

Neurofibromatosis

Macrocephaly unrelated to either tumor or aqueductal stenosis is common in children with neurofibromatosis.

MICROCEPHALY

Microcephaly is defined as two standard deviations below the mean. Most, but not all, patients with microcephaly are retarded or have learning disabilities. Rarely, patients with microcephaly are seen that have normal intellect.

Primary Microcephaly Unrelated to Acquired Causes

- Genetic: microcephaly vera
- Markedly decreased head circumference that is more than four standard deviations below the mean
- Mostly dominant
- May be recessive or X-linked
- Receding forehead
- Pointed vertex
- Depletion of neurons in layers two and three of the cerebral cortex

Secondary or Acquired Microcephaly

- Intrauterine causes
  - Drugs, alcohol
  - Ionizing radiation
  - Maternal malnutrition
  - Diabetes
  - Immuno and organic aminoacidopathies
  - Toxoplasmosis, cytomegalovirus, rubella, herpes simplex, and human immunodeficiency virus
- Degenerative disease
- Pelizaeus-Merzbacher disease
- Batten disease (neuronal ceroid lipofuscinosis)
- Down syndrome
- Craniosynostosis
- Rett syndrome

Suggested Reading

Aicardi J. The agyria-pachygyria complex: a spectrum of cortical malformations. *Brain Dev* 1991;13:1–8.

Aronyk KE. The history and classification of hydrocephalus. *Neurosurg Clin North Am* 1993;4:599–609.

Book JA, Schut JW, Reed AC. A clinical and genetical study of microcephaly. *Am J Ment Defic* 1953;57:637–660.

Cole TR, Hughes HE. Autosomal dominant macrocephaly: benign familial macrocephaly or a new syndrome? *Am J Med Genet* 1991;41:115–124.

De Meyer W. Classification of cerebral malformations. *Birth defects original article series* 1971;7:78–93.

Dobyns WB, Elias ER, Newlin AC, et al. Causal heterogeneity in isolated lissencephaly. *Neurology* 1992;42:1375–1388.

Dolk H. The predictive value of microcephaly during the first year of life for mental retardation at seven years. *Dev Med Child Neurol* 1991;33:974–983.

Gooskens RH, Willemse J, Bijlsma JB, Hanlo PW. Megalencephaly: definition and classification. *Brain Dev* 1988;10:1–7.

Guiffre R, Pastore FS, De Santis S. Connatal (fetal) hydrocephalus: an acquired pathology? *Childs Nerv Syst* 1995;11:97–101.

Harding B, Copp AJ. Malformations. In: Graham DI, Lantos PL, eds. *Greenfield's neuropathology*, 6th ed. New York: Oxford University Press, 1997:417–422.

Jacobson RI. Abnormalities of the skull in children. *Neurol Clin* 1985; 3:117–145.

Little JR, Houser OW, MacCarty CS. Clinical manifestations of aqueductal stenosis in adults. *J Neurosurg* 1975;43:546–552.

Loebstein R, Koren G. Pregnancy outcome and neurodevelopment of children exposed in utero to psychoactive drugs: the Motherisk experience. *J Psychiatry Neurosci* 1997;22:192–196.

McKusick VA. *Mendelian inheritance in man: a catalog of human genes and genetic disorders,* 11th ed. Baltimore: Johns Hopkins University Press, 1994.

Steinlin M, Zurrer M, Martin E, et al. Contribution of magnetic resonance imaging on the evaluation of microcephaly. *Neuropediatrics* 1991;22:184–189.

Volpe JJ. *Neurology of the newborn.* Philadelphia: WB Saunders, 1995.

Wisniewski K, Bambska M, Sher JH, et al. A clinical neuropathological study of the fetal alcohol syndrome. *Neuropediatrics* 1983;14:197–201.

Chapter 26

Brain Tumors

Case

A 2-year-old child presents with a 3-week history of early morning headache and vomiting. On examination, she has a large head (51 cm) with papilledema, right sixth nerve palsy, and truncal ataxia. Magnetic resonance imaging (MRI) reveals a large enhancing heterogeneous mass in the vermis of the cerebellum that is occluding the fourth ventricle.

Diagnosis

Medulloblastoma

Brain tumors have an **incidence of approximately 3 per 100,000 children**, with a **peak from the ages of 5 to 9 years**. Brian tumors are the most common solid tumor and the second most common malignancy in children. Signs and symptoms vary depending on the location, the neurologic system with which the tumor interferes, and the age of the child.

NONLOCALIZING SIGNS AND SYMPTOMS THAT REFLECT INCREASING INTRACRANIAL PRESSURE

Symptoms

- Irritability
- Personality change
- Headache

- Vomiting: especially in the early morning or during sleep
- Diplopia (may or may not be localizing): usually sixth nerve palsy

Signs

- An increase in head circumference
- Papilledema (may have a larger blind spot)
- Head tilt
  - Incipient tonsillar herniation
  - Fourth nerve palsy
- Sixth nerve paresis (inability to abduct the eye fully on lateral gaze)

LOCALIZING SIGNS AND SYMPTOMS

Posterior Fossa: Cerebellum

General

- Appendicular ataxia
- Truncal ataxia
- Scanning speech
- Pendular reflexes
- Hypotonia
- Slow coarse nystagmus to the side of the lesion
- Early signs: increased intracranial pressure (ICP)

Examples of Cerebellar Tumors

Medulloblastoma

- Malignant
- Usually midline (vermis cerebellum)
- Truncal ataxia
- Early signs: increased ICP
- MRI
  - Heterogeneous enhancing mass with obstructive hydrocephalus
  - Disseminates in the cerebrospinal fluid (CSF)
  - Occasional extraneural metastases
- Treatment
  - Maximal surgical resection

- Craniospinal radiation (except for children less than 3 years of age)
- Adjuvant chemotherapy

- Survival rates (if gross total resection and no metastases): higher than 70% to 80%

Cerebellar Astrocytoma

- Peak incidence from 5 to 14 years of age
- Juvenile pilocytic astrocytoma (low grade)
- Usually hemispheric: may be midline
- Localized disease: usually a cyst with a mural nodule
- Presents with cerebellar signs and increased ICP
- Appendicular ataxia
- MRI: cyst with enhancing rim or mural nodule
- Treatment: maximal surgical resection
- Prognosis: more than 90% survival if totally removed

Ependymoma

- Location: fourth ventricle, although may occur in lateral or third ventricles and may even be unrelated to the ventricular system
- Peak incidence: birth to 5 years of age
- Early increase in ICP; ataxia
- MRI and computed tomography: calcified hyperdense mass with obstructive hydrocephalus; may extrude through the foramina of Luschka and Magendie and wrap around brainstem
- Disseminates in the CSF late in the course of the illness
- Treatment
    - Maximal surgical resection
    - Local radiation
    - Chemotherapy, especially if tumor has not been completely resected
- Survival rates: 30% to 50%; best survival rates (60%) if gross total resection

Brainstem

General Features

- Cranial neuropathies
- Long tract signs (hemiparesis)
- Cerebellar signs: ataxia
- Late development of increased ICP

Example of Brainstem Tumor: Brainstem Glioma

- Peak incidence: 5 to 14 years of age
- Highly malignant (glioblastoma)
- Worst prognosis if it is localized to the pons
- Better prognosis if it is cervicomedullary, focal, cystic, or exophytic
- Treatment
  - Local radiation (palliative)
  - Chemotherapy (unproven)
- Prognosis: uniformly fatal if its location is the pontine

Cerebral Hemisphere

General Features

- Seizures: partial, both with and without secondary generalization
- Hemiparesis
- Sensory disturbance
- Visual field defects
- Aphasia
- Decline in school performance

Examples of Cerebral Hemisphere Tumors

Low-Grade Astrocytoma

- Long duration of symptoms
- Seizures: common
- Localized disease with lateralizing signs
- Hypodense on computed tomography; hypointense on MRI—may enhance
- Treatment
  - Surgery
  - Radiation necessary at recurrence
- Prognosis: more than 70% have 5-year survival rates

Anaplastic Astrocytomas and/or Glioblastoma Multiforme

- Rapidly progressive
- Highly malignant
- CSF dissemination seen late in course
- Lateralizing signs
- Increased ICP
- MRI: mass effect, edema, ring enhancement

- Treatment
  - Maximal surgical resection
  - Local radiation (wide ports)
  - Chemotherapy
- Prognosis: 5-year survival rate of approximately 30% for anaplastic astrocytoma; 5-year survival rate of approximately 10% for glioblastoma multiforme

Primitive Neuroectodermal Tumors

- Rapidly progressive
- Highly malignant
- Disseminate in the CSF
- Occasional extraneural metastases
- MRI
  - Large mass without peritumoral edema
  - Cysts plus hemorrhage
  - Enhancement
- Treatment
  - Maximal surgical resection
  - Craniospinal radiation
  - Chemotherapy
- Prognosis: survival rates of 30% to 40%

Midline Tumors

General Features

- Optic atrophy
- Visual loss
- Nystagmus
- Endocrinopathies (either increase or decrease in appetite, precocious puberty)
- Hydrocephalus
- Personality change

Examples of Midline Tumors

Optic Gliomas

- Juvenile pilocytic astrocytoma
- Associated with neurofibromatosis, type 1
- Decreased visual acuity: nystagmus (chiasm)

- Mostly indolent, but may be aggressive
- Treatment
  - Radiation in older children if progressive
  - Chemotherapy for children less than 5 years of age if progressive
- Prognosis: prolonged survival (better in children with neurofibromatosis)

Craniopharyngiomas

- Onset in latter half of first decade or early part of second decade
- Usually suprasellar
- Can fill the cavity of the third ventricle and expand to involve the visual pathways and hypothalamus
- Cystic or partially solid with a capsule
- Increased ICP and visual defects (usually asymmetric)
- Endocrinopathies
- Computed tomography and/or MRI: calcified cystic mass
- Treatment
  - Surgery
  - Radiation if less than gross total removal
- After surgery, may have diabetes insipidus and/or other endocrinopathies
- Long-term survival but with frequent recurrence

BENIGN TUMORS

- Dysembryoblastic neuroepithelial tumor
- Ganglioglioma
- Oligodendroglioma
- Central neurocytoma
- Meningioma
- Pleomorphic xanthoastrocytoma
- Subependymal giant cell astrocytoma

LONG-TERM EFFECTS OF RADIATION THERAPY

Decreased Intelligence (Progressive)

Risk factors for decreased intelligence include young age, large volume radiation (whole brain), high dose radiation, the location of tumor, the concomitant use of methotrexate, the presence of vasculopathy and leukoencephalopathy, and perioperative complications.

Endocrinopathies

Endocrinopathies that may result from radiation therapy include the following:

- Growth hormone deficiency: seen in 80% of children receiving whole brain radiation; may occur with radiation to the posterior fossa alone if the ventromedian nucleus of the hypothalamus is included in the radiation port
- Short stature
  - Growth hormone deficiency
  - Spinal shortening
    - Poor spinal growth after spinal radiation
    - Worse in young children
- Hypothyroidism
  - Primary (decrease in thyroxine, increase in thyroid-stimulating hormone): due to radiation of the thyroid gland as part of craniospinal radiation
  - Secondary (decreased in thyroxine and in thyroid-stimulating hormone): less common, due to direct radiation effect on pituitary gland (thyroid-stimulating hormone)
- Gonadal dysfunction
  - Spinal radiation: may cause ovarian dysfunction
  - Cyclophosphamide: may cause gonadal dysfunction in males

Second Malignancies

- Reported after both low and high dose radiation therapy
- Include meningiomas, high grade astrocytomas
- Typically aggressive
- May occur after chemotherapy in the absence of radiation
  - Etoposide, cyclophosphamide, or cisplatin
  - Acute myelogenous leukemia, myelodysplastic syndrome

Suggested Reading

Adamson TE, Wiestler OD, Kleihues P, et al. Correlation of clinical and pathological features in surgically treated craniopharyngiomas. *J Neurosurg* 1990;73:12–17.

Albright AL, Wisoff JH, Zeltzer P, et al. Prognostic factors in children with supratentorial (nonpineal) primitive neuroectodermal tumors. *Pediatr Neurosurg* 1995;22:1–7.

Ashwal S, Hinshaw DB Jr, Bedros A. CNS primitive neuroectodermal tumors of childhood. *Med Pediatr Oncol* 1984;12:180–188.

Burger PC, Green SB. Patient age, histologic features, and length of survival in patients with glioblastoma multiforme. *Cancer* 1987;59:1617–1625.

Chintagumpala M, Berg S, Blaney SM. Treatment controversies in medulloblastoma. *Curr Opin Oncol* 2001;13:154–159.

Cohen ME, Duffner PK. *Brain tumors in children: principles of diagnosis and treatment,* 2nd ed. New York: Raven Press, 1994.

Duffner PK, Krischer JP, Sanford RA, et al. Prognostic factors in infants and very young children with intracranial ependymomas. *Pediatr Neurosurg* 1998;28:215–222.

Epstein F. Intrinsic brain stem tumors of childhood. Surgical indications. In: Homburger F, ed. *Progress in experimental tumor research.* Basel, Switzerland: S Karger, 1987:160–169.

Fisher PG, Tontiplaphol A, Pearlman EM, et al. Childhood cerebellar hemangioblastoma does not predict germline or somatic mutations in the Von Hippel-Lindau tumor suppressor gene. *Ann Neurol* 2002;51:257–260.

Freeman CR, Krischer J, Sanford RA, et al. Hyperfractionated radiation therapy in brain stem tumors: results of treatment at the 7020 cGy dose level of Pediatric Oncology Group study 8495. *Cancer* 1991;68:474–481.

Gilles FH, Sobel E, Leviton A, et al. Epidemiology of seizures in children with brain tumors. *Neurooncology* 1992;12:53–68.

Gjerris F, Klinken L. Long-term prognosis of children with benign cerebellar astrocytoma. *J Neurosurg* 1978;49:179–184.

Goldwein JW, Leahy JM, Packer RJ, et al. Intracranial ependymomas in children. *Int J Radiat Oncol Biol Phys* 1990;19:1497–1502.

Hetelekidis S, Barnes PD, Tao ML, et al. 20-year experience in childhood craniopharyngioma. *Int J Radiat Oncol Biol Phys* 1993;27:189–195.

Hirsch JF, Rose C, Pierre-Kahn A, et al. Benign astrocytic and oligodendrocytic tumors of the cerebral hemispheres in children. *J Neurosurg* 1989;70:568–572.

Jenkin D, Shabanah MA, Shail EA, et al. Prognostic factors for medulloblastoma. *Int J Radiat Oncol Biol Phys* 2000;47:573–584.

Johnson JH, Hariharan S, Berman J, et al. Clinical outcome of pediatric gangliogliomas: ninety-nine cases over 20 years. *Pediatr Neurosurg* 1997;27:203–207.

Mahoney DH, Cohen MR, Friedman HS, et al. Carboplatin is effective therapy for young children with progressive optic pathway tumors: a Pediatric Oncology Group phase II study. *Neurooncology* 2000;2:213–220.

Packer RJ, Cogen P, Vezina G, et al. Medulloblastoma: clinical and biologic aspects [Review]. *Neurooncology* 1999;1:232–250.

Chapter 27

Neurologic Complications of Leukemia

Case

A 5-year-old girl has been treated for the last 2 years for acute lymphocytic leukemia. She had received both intravenous and intrathecal methotrexate as part of her treatment regimen. She now presents with seizures, dementia, and motor abnormalities. Computed tomography revealed calcification in the basal ganglia, increased ventricular size, and evidence of cerebral atrophy. Magnetic resonance imaging revealed increased T2-weighted signals extending to the gray–white matter border.

Diagnosis

Methotrexate-induced leukoencephalopathy

MENINGEAL LEUKEMIA

- Leukemic cell involvement, primarily of the arachnoid
- Headache, vomiting, papilledema, and nuchal rigidity
  - Increased intracranial pressure
  - Communicating hydrocephalus
    - Leukemic cells block the resorption of cerebrospinal fluid into the arachnoid villi
    - Lumbar puncture: increased opening pressure, blasts, increased protein levels, decreased glucose levels
- Seizures
- Cranial neuropathies: II, VI, VII, VIII

STROKE

Strokes are seen in 4% of children with acute lymphoblastic leukemia. Most occur within the first year of treatment or in relapse.

Hemorrhagic Stroke

- Decreased platelets
- Trauma in the presence of decreased levels of platelets
- Disseminated intravascular coagulation
- Rapid increase in white blood cells to more than 100,000 mm^3 at presentation
- L-Asparaginase—may lead to decreased fibrinogen
- Chloromas: may compress blood vessels

Thrombotic Stroke

- Increase in white blood cells
- Complications caused by L-asparaginase: secondary to decreased levels of antithrombin 3, plasminogen, and protein C
- Central nervous system (CNS) infection, especially fungal (arterial)
- Venous stroke (bacterial)
- Dehydration
- Dural sinus thrombosis
    - Leukemic infiltration sinus
    - L-Asparaginase

HYPOTHALAMIC SYNDROME

- Infiltration of hypothalamus by leukemic cells
- Hyperphagia with obesity
- Headache
- Vomiting
- Increased intracranial pressure

SEIZURES

General

- Seen in 4% to 13% of patients
- Partial, both with and without secondary generalization

Etiologies

- Vascular
  - Hemorrhage secondary to decrease in platelets and disseminated intravascular coagulation
  - Stroke
- Infectious: meningitis or encephalitis; origin can be bacterial, viral, or fungal
- Metabolic
  - Decrease in sodium secondary to a syndrome of inappropriate secretion of antidiuretic hormone (SIADH) after administration of cisplatin and vincristine
  - Decreased blood sugar and decreased calcium and magnesium levels
- Rapid cell lysis
- Methotrexate: can provoke an acute reaction
- Leukoencephalopathy: causes seizures, dementia, and motor abnormalities
- Narcotics and antiemetics: may decrease the seizure threshold

PERIPHERAL NEUROPATHY SECONDARY TO CHEMOTHERAPY

The incidence of this is related to the dose and duration of therapy.

Vincristine Neuropathy

- Distal symmetric sensory motor neuropathy
- Interruption of axoplasmic transport
- Complete recovery usually seen by 4 months after the completion of treatment
- Increased risk for severe neurotoxicity in the following:
  - Infants, young children, adolescents
  - Cachectic patients
  - Patients confined to bedrest
  - Those with underlying peripheral neuropathy (e.g., Charcot-Marie-Tooth disease)

Thalidomide Neuropathy

- Sensory neuropathy
- Paresthesias and numbness in a stocking–glove distribution
- Individual may not recover

Cisplatin Neuropathy

- Sensory peripheral neuropathy
- Severe neurotoxicity resolves; paresthesias may persist

Paclitaxel

- Distal sensory neuropathy
- Reversible
- Dose dependent

LEUKOENCEPHALOPATHY

- Associated with cranial irradiation with or without methotrexate
- Risk increased if intrathecal methotrexate is given in the face of CNS leukemia or communicating hydrocephalus. Decreased clearance of methotrexate causes increased levels and prolonged duration of exposure of the brain to the methotrexate
- May occur with intravenous or intrathecal methotrexate in the absence of cranial irradiation or CNS leukemia
- Pathology
    - Loss of oligodendroglia
    - Mineralizing microangiopathy
    - Dystrophic calcification
    - White matter necrosis
- Computed tomography
    - Calcification of the basal ganglia
    - Hypodense areas
    - Widened subarachnoid spaces
- Magnetic resonance imaging
    - Increase in T2-weighted signals extending from the ventricles to the gray matter–white matter junction
    - Best seen on flair sequence
- Clinical signs
    - Dementia
    - Focal motor signs
    - Seizures
    - Ataxia
- Death or severe neurologic disability

MYELOPATHY INDUCED BY CHEMOTHERAPY

- May follow the use of intrathecal methotrexate, with or without the administration of intrathecal cytosine arabinoside

- Increased risk in children with meningeal disease: leads to increased methotrexate levels and prolonged duration of exposure of the brain to the methotrexate in the CSF

Clinical Signs

- Paraplegia or paraparesis
- Sensory level: inability to feel pain and temperature below a certain level
- Loss of bowel and bladder control

Differential Diagnosis

- Cord compression
  - Epidural hematoma
    - Trauma
    - Lumbar puncture in the presence of decreased platelets
  - Tumor: chloroma
  - Epidural abscess
- Transverse myelitis

Prognosis

- Poor
- No effective therapy

SPINAL CORD COMPRESSION

- Epidural tumor infiltration
  - Back pain
  - Weakness in the lower extremities
  - Incontinence
  - Sensory level: inability to feel pain and temperature below a certain level
  - Usually thoracic lumbar
  - Magnetic resonance imaging: may be diagnostic
  - Cerebrospinal fluid protein: increased
  - Treatment: local radiation therapy and dexamethasone
- Hematoma (epidural or subdural)
  - Lumbar puncture in the face of low platelets
  - Trauma in the face of low platelets
  - Evacuate clot

INFECTION

- Bacterial meningitis
- Viral and/or encephalitis

  - Herpes
  - Varicella
  - Rubella
  - *Toxoplasma gondii*
- Fungal meningitis: *Cryptococcus*
- Brain abscess: *Aspergillosis*, mucormycosis, candida, nocardia

LYMPHOMA: NON-HODGKIN

- CNS involvement in 5% to 11% of patients
- Leptomeningeal metastases
  - Cranial nerve palsies in II, VI, VII
  - Focal motor or sensory dysfunction
  - Headache, nausea, and vomiting
  - Radiculopathy
- Spinal epidural disease
  - Cord compression: growth of tumor through the intervertebral foramina into the epidural space
  - Compression fractures of the vertebral bodies
  - Lymphomatous expansion of the vertebral bodies
  - Treatment: laminectomy if acute deterioration is present; radiation and/or chemotherapy

Suggested Reading

Duffner PK, Cohen ME, Berger P, et al. Abnormalities of computed tomography scans and altered methotrexate clearance in children with central nervous system leukemia. *Ann Neurol* 1981;10:286–287.

Feinberg WM, Swenson MR. Cerebrovascular complications of L-asparaginase therapy. *Neurol* 1988;38:127–133.

Keidan SE. Paraplegia in childhood malignant disease. *Acta Paediatr Scand* 1967;172:110–118.

Mahoney D, Shuster J, Nitschke R. Acute neurotoxicity in children with B-precursor acute lymphoid leukemia: an association with intermediate-dose intravenous methotrexate and intrathecal triple therapy. A Pediatric Oncology Group study. *J Clin Oncol* 1998;16:1712–1722.

Maytal J, Grossman R, Yusuf FH, et al. Prognosis and treatment of seizures in children with acute lymphoblastic leukemia. *Epilepsia* 1995;36:831–836.

Ochs JJ, Bowman P, Pui CH, et al. Seizures in childhood lymphoblastic leukemia patients. *Lancet* 1984;2:1422–1424.

Price RA, Jamieson PA. The central nervous system in childhood leukemia. *Cancer* 1975;35:306–318.

Chapter 28

Pseudotumor Cerebri

Case

A 13-year-old obese girl presents with a 3-week history of headache and vomiting. Over the past week, she has developed double vision. She was taking tetracycline for acne. On examination, she has papilledema, normal visual acuity, and a left sixth nerve palsy. Her neurologic examination is otherwise normal. Magnetic resonance imaging and magnetic resonance venography (MRV) are normal. Lumbar puncture reveals an opening pressure of 450 mm H_2O with normal protein and glucose levels and a normal cell count.

Diagnosis

Pseudotumor cerebri (idiopathic intracranial hypertension)

Pseudotumor cerebri is defined as a diffuse increase in intracranial pressure in the presence of normal cerebrospinal fluid and normal brain imaging.

SYMPTOMS

- Headache: increases with Valsalva maneuver
- Vomiting
- Diplopia
- Visual obscuration

In *young children,* the following are also seen:

- Somnolence and irritability
- Bulging fontanelle

SIGNS

- Papilledema
  - Increase in blind spot
  - Normal visual acuity (initially)
- Sixth nerve palsy: nonlateralizing

RISK FACTORS

- Girls: adolescent and obese
- Drugs
  - Tetracycline
  - Birth control pills
  - Vitamin A: increased or decreased
  - Steroid withdrawal
- Endocrinopathy
  - Treatment with growth hormone
  - Treatment with thyroid hormone
  - Hyperthyroidism
  - Adrenal insufficiency or hyperadrenalism
  - Hypoparathyroidism
- Refeeding in malnourished children and those with cystic fibrosis
- Iron deficiency anemia

DIFFERENTIAL DIAGNOSIS

- Mass lesion
- Hydrocephalus
- Lateral sinus thrombosis
  - Mastoiditis
  - Otitis media
- Sagittal sinus thrombosis
  - Systemic lupus erythematosus
  - Polycythemia

- Dehydration
- Hypercoagulable states
- Malignancy
  - Carcinomatosis
  - Gliomatosis cerebri
  - Leukemia

EVALUATION

- Magnetic resonance imaging of the brain
  - Normal
  - Small ventricles: may or may not be present
  - Effacement of cortical sulci: may or may not be present
- MRV: assess flow in lateral and sagittal sinus
- Visual acuity and visual fields: repeat frequently
- Lumbar puncture
  - Increased opening pressure (greater than 200 mm H_2O)
  - Normal protein and glucose levels, normal cell count

TREATMENT

- Relieve pressure to preserve vision
- Lumbar puncture
  - Reduce pressure to half the opening pressure
  - Remove 10 to 20 mL cerebrospinal fluid, but not below 200 mm H_2O
- Acetazolamide
  - Dose of 10 to 20 mg per kg per day
  - Can range from 250 mg twice daily to 500 mg twice daily
- Failure of lumbar puncture and acetazolamide—try the following:
  - Decadron, 12 mg per m^2 for 2 weeks, *OR*
  - Prednisone, 2 mg per kg (maximum of 60 mg) for 2 weeks
- Failure of the above—try the following:
  - Optic nerve fenestration, *OR*
  - Lumboperitoneal shunt
    - May cause acquired Chiari malformation
    - May cause tethered cord

If this condition is left untreated, the increased intracranial pressure may cause optic atrophy and permanent visual loss.

Suggested Reading

Babikian P, Corbett J, Bell W. Idiopathic intracranial hypertension in children: the Iowa experience. *J Child Neurol* 1994;9:144–149.

Corbett JJ, Savino PJ, Thompson HS, et al. Visual loss in pseudotumor cerebri. Follow up of 57 patients from 5 to 41 years and a profile of 14 patients with permanent severe visual loss. *Arch Neurol* 1982;39:461–474.

Jacobson DM, Karanjia PM, Olson KA, Warner JJ. Computed tomography ventricular size has a predictive value in diagnosing pseudotumor cerebri. *Neurology* 1990;40:1454–1455.

Johnston I, Paterson A. Benign intracranial hypertension. I. Diagnosis and prognosis. *Brain* 1974;97:289–300.

Soler D, Cox T, Bullock P, et al. Diagnosis and management of benign intracranial hypertension. *Arch Dis Child* 1998;78:89–94.

Chapter 29

Loss of Consciousness

Case

An agitated and delirious 3-year-old boy is brought to the emergency room. He has no focal signs on neurologic examination. His pupils react to light. Fundi are normal. No evidence suggests the presence of increased intracranial pressure, and no localizing neurologic signs are found. His past medical history is unremarkable. The family history reveals that the mother is a manic-depressive and that she is on a number of psycholeptic agents.

Diagnosis

Acute drug intoxication

A clue to a nonintracranial cause of coma is the normal neurologic examination. No evidence of increased intracranial pressure was seen, and the pupils reacted normally to light.

Loss of consciousness is loosely defined as unawareness of self and the environment. A normal state of consciousness requires an arousal system, a sleep–wake cycle, and intact autonomic and vegetative brain function.

IMPORTANT DEFINITIONS

- Hallucinations: false sensory perception without an external basis in fact.
- Illusion: false sensory perception with an external basis in fact.

- Delusion: thought disorder out of keeping with a person's background, culture, religion, or education.
- Delirium: agitation, disorientation, and a hypermotor state with or without hallucinations and/or illusions.
- Confusion: inattentiveness, dullness of perception, and disorientation, initially to time and then to place and person. The more significant the disorientation is, the more severe the problem.
- Lethargy: reduced wakefulness and level of alertness. Can be easily aroused.
- Obtundation: sleepy, difficult to arouse.
- Stupor: arousable only with vigorous stimulation.
- Coma: Unarousable despite stimulation.
- Vegetative state: unawareness of self and the environment with preservation of autonomic functions. Wake–sleep cycles are maintained.
- Locked-in syndrome: cognition and awareness are preserved, but all volitional movements are absent or are severely limited.

COMMON CAUSES OF ALTERATION IN CONSCIOUSNESS

- Central nervous system (CNS) etiology (20% to 30% of cases)
  - Trauma
  - Infection of the nervous system
  - Neoplasms
  - Cerebrovascular disease
  - Seizures
- Non-CNS etiology (70% to 80% of cases)
  - Cardiovascular abnormalities: syncope (vasovagal or vagalvaso)
  - Drugs: toxins
  - Endocrine: hypoglycemia
  - High fever: temperature greater than 40.6°C (105°F)
  - Hypoxic ischemic abnormalities
    - Drowning
    - Carbon monoxide intoxication
  - Metabolic: acidosis, electrolyte abnormalities (i.e., calcium, sodium, or potassium)
  - Non-CNS infection

CLUES TO ETIOLOGY

- General examination: assess vital functions (i.e., respiration, blood pressure, pulse, and temperature)

- Look for signs of trauma
  - Raccoon's eye: periorbital ecchymosis
  - Battle sign (i.e., blood behind the mastoid): basilar skull fracture
  - Cerebrospinal fluid leak from the nose or ear
- Rashes
  - Meningococcemia
    - Purpuric
    - Hemorrhagic lesions of the skin
  - Rickettsial infection: rash on the hands and feet
- Abnormal odor
  - Alcohol
  - Ketoacidosis
  - Uremia
  - Hepatic coma
- Neurologic examination
  - May be localizing
  - Papilledema: suggests increased intracranial pressure
  - Doll's eyes (oculocephalic reflex)
    - Present in patient with intact brainstem
    - Asymmetric doll's eyes: suggests brainstem abnormality
  - Meningeal irritation: suggests blood or infection
  - Intact pupillary responses
    - Etiology usually metabolic or drugs, rather than a primary CNS cause
    - Rule out cycloplegic drugs (i.e., atropine), other anticholinergics, or sympathomimetic agents
- Herniation: size of pupils, type of respiration, pulse, blood pressure, and tone all suggest the degree of herniation

HEAD TRAUMA

Most head trauma in children is minor, and it does not require treatment other than observation. However, each year preventable head trauma is a significant cause of death in children. The Glasgow coma scale (GCS) is commonly used to evaluate the severity of the head trauma (see Appendix VI).

Mild Head Trauma

- GCS score: 13 to 15
- Loss of consciousness for less than 30 minutes

- No neurologic damage
- No evidence of skull fracture (i.e., depressed skull fracture)

Moderate Head Trauma

- GCS score: 9 to 12
- Loss of consciousness of variable length
- Focal neurologic deficit
- Depressed skull fracture
- Intracranial bleed: may or may not be present

Severe Head Trauma

- GCS score: less than 8
- Prolonged loss of consciousness
- Focal neurologic deficit
- Intracranial trauma: bleeding or axonal injury
- Depressed skull fracture

Concussion

This is defined as loss of consciousness, no matter how brief. The practice parameters of the American Academy of Neurology for the management of concussions in sports are the current standards used in the United States for evaluation of minor concussion in children (see Appendix VII).

CENTRAL NERVOUS SYSTEM HERNIATION

Herniation is the movement of the brain from an area of high resistance to an area of lower resistance. With supratentorial herniation, the brain moves toward and through the foramen magnum in a cephalocaudal fashion. In transtentorial herniation, the uncus, the leading edge of the temporal lobe, herniates across the tentorium toward the foramen magnum, compressing the more medial adjacent structures (i.e., nerves, vessels, and brainstem), again in a cephalocaudal fashion.

Signs of Herniation

Pupils

- The pupils become progressively smaller as herniation progresses in a caudal fashion, until the patient is agonal and the pupils dilate.

- Light reflex is lost, except in cases of metabolic coma (rule out the use of cycloplegic drugs).
- Doll's eye reflex (eyes move in the opposite direction the head is turned) is seen in the comatose patient with an intact brainstem, and it becomes asymmetric and ultimately is absent with the progressive loss of brainstem function.

Motor Response

- Subcortical: purposeful movement to painful stimulation
- Diencephalon: decorticate flexion of the arms and extension of the leg
- Midbrain: decerebration extension of the arms and legs
- Pons and medullary: flaccid limbs

Vital Signs

- Subcortical and diencephalic: Cheyne-Stokes breathing
- Mesencephalic: central neurogenic hyperventilation
- Upper pons: apneustic respirations (i.e., short rapid respirations superimposed upon a large inspiratory effort)
- Pons and medulla: ataxic respirations (i.e., gasping, irregular breaths)
- Cushing reflex (signs of incipient herniation): increased systolic blood pressure; diastolic pressure is variable; wide pulse pressure; bradycardia

Treatment

- Support the "ABCs"
  - Airway
  - Breathing
  - Circulation
- Treat the suspected infection
- Correct acid-base abnormalities
- Administer glucose
- Manage agitation
- Treat seizures if present
- With signs of herniation
  - Immediate neurosurgical consultation
  - Consider mannitol in dose of 0.5 to 2 g per kg
  - Hyperventilation to decrease intracranial pressure
  - Limit fluids to two-thirds of maintenance

Suggested Reading

Adelson PD, Kochanek PM. Head injuries in children. *J Child Neurol* 1998; 13:2–15.

Adelson PK, Clyde B, Kochanek PM, et al. Cerebrovascular response in infants and young children following severe traumatic brain injury: a preliminary report. *Pediatr Neurosurg* 1997;26:200–207.

Bruce DA, Alavi A, Bilaniuk L, et al. Diffuse cerebral swelling following head injuries in children. The syndrome of "malignant brain edema." *J Neurosurg* 1981;54:170–178.

Craft AW, Shaw DA, Cartlidge NE. Head injuries in children. *BMJ* 1972; 4:200–203.

Ellenhorn MJ, Schonwald S, Ordog G, Wasserberger J, eds. *Medical toxicology: diagnosis and treatment of human poisoning.* Baltimore: Williams & Wilkins, 1997.

Kulberg A. Substance abuse: clinical identification and management. *Pediatr Clin North Am* 1986;33:325–361.

Kurlan R. Tourette's syndrome and "PANDAS": will the relation bear out? Pediatric autoimmune neuropsychiatric disorders associated with streptococcal infection. *Neurology* 1998;50:1530–1534.

McClain PW, Sacks JJ, Froehlke RG, Ewigman BG. Estimates of fatal child abuse and neglect. United States, 1979 through 1988. *Pediatrics* 1993;91: 338–343.

Mitchell AA, Lovejoy FH, Goldman P. Drug ingestions associated with miosis in comatose children. *J Pediatr* 1976;89:303–305.

Pearn J, Nixon J, Ansford A, Corcoran A. Accidental poisoning in childhood. Five year urban population study with 15 year analysis of fatality. *Br Med J (Clin Res Ed)* 1984;288:44–46.

Plum FB, Posner JB. *Diagnosis of stupor and coma,* 3rd ed. Philadelphia: FA Davis, 1980.

Chapter 30

Gait

Case

A 12-year-old boy presents to the office with the inability to walk unassisted. He tends to sway from the waist. He has a wide-based stance that does not increase his stability. As the youngster walks, he tends to lurch and stagger. The rest of the neurologic examination is unremarkable. The family history indicates that the parents have been recently divorced. The mother works every day, and the child is primarily cared for by a teenaged baby-sitter.

Diagnosis

Astasia-abasia
The patient was referred for psychiatric counseling.

A gait disorder refers to alteration in ambulation from any cause. Ataxia refers to disorders in coordination resulting from errors in timing, rate, and duration of movement. In children, gait abnormalities may be either developmental or acquired. Most children initiate walking between 9 and 18 months of age. Even in the presence of significant development delay, in the absence of structural abnormalities, most children eventually walk. Some may be constitutionally awkward, and they may never develop the skills associated with hopping, skipping, or riding a two-wheeler. These children may be intellectually delayed yet may have no other neurologic abnormalities. Acquired gait disorders, on the other hand, may have their source in a variety of structural and anatomic defects.

Gait disorders may result from abnormalities of the upper motor neuron, cerebellum, and peripheral nervous system, or they may be musculoskeletal in origin (e.g., cortical stroke, cerebellar tumor, diabetic neuropathy, and muscular dystrophy).

UPPER MOTOR NEURON LESION

- This lesion involves both pyramidal and extrapyramidal motor systems.
- The arm contralateral to the lesion tends to be flexed at the elbow and at the wrist.
- Decreased arm swing is seen when walking. The involved leg is circumducted.
- The patient may drift to the involved side. Depending on the degree of extrapyramidal involvement, associated dystonia (abnormal attitude of posture), chorea, or ballistic movements may be present.
- Reflexes are increased.
- Tone is increased.
- The Babinski sign is readily obtained.

FRONTAL APRAXIA

- Inability to initiate movement
- Small, quick steps
- Stooped posture
- Decreased associated movements
- Increased reflexes

SENSORY ATAXIA

- High stepping gait secondary to proprioceptive loss
- Seen in thalamic lesions or lesions of the dorsal column

CEREBELLAR ATAXIA

- This is characterized by a wide-based gait and an inability to turn on a narrow base.
- The involvement of the midline structures is associated with truncal instability.

- The involvement of the lateral cerebellar structures is associated with limb ataxia, dysmetria, and dysdiadochokinesis.
- Tremor is perpendicular to the line of movement.
- Reflexes are pendular.
- Tone is decreased.

PERIPHERAL NERVOUS SYSTEM: ROOT OR NERVE LESIONS

- Foot drop
- Loss of reflexes
- Sensory loss
- Distal weakness
- Gait: high steppage associated with a bilateral foot drop
- Absent reflexes
- Decreased sensation

MUSCULOSKELETAL ORIGIN

- Gait is waddling.
- Arm movement is decreased.
- When the child walks, the shoulders and arms are supinated, rather than being held in a semisupinated position.
- Reflexes are preserved.
- The child has more difficulty going down stairs than up stairs.
- Weakness is proximal rather than distal.

FUNCTIONAL

Astasia-abasia

- The child sways from the waist.
- The wide-based stance does not increase stability.
- The child lurches and staggers.
- Strength, tone, sensation, and deep tendon reflexes are normal.
- Secondary gain may be apparent.

Camptocormia

- Flexed posture
- Inability to walk upright
- No anatomic abnormality

Antalgic Gait

In antalgic gait, limitation of movement is secondary to pain in the spine, hip, or long bone.

Suggested Reading

Burnett CN, Johnson EW. Development of gait in childhood. I. Method *Dev Med Child Neurol* 1971;13:196–206.

Burnett CN, Johnson EW. Development of gait in childhood. II. *Dev Med Child Neurol* 1971;13:207–215.

Fenichel GM. *Clinical pediatric neurology: a signs and symptoms approach,* 4th ed. Philadelphia: WB Saunders, 2001.

Norlin R, Odenrick P, Sandlund B. Development of gait in normal children. *J Pediatr Orthop* 1981;1:261–266.

Swaiman KF. Muscular tone and gait disturbances. In: Swaiman KF, Ashwal S, eds. *Pediatric neurology: principles and practice,* 3rd ed. Vol. 1. St. Louis: Mosby, 1999.

Chapter 31

Cerebellar Ataxia

Case

A 2-year-old girl presents to the hospital with a 3-day history of inability to sit, chaotic movement of the eyes, and profound truncal ataxia. The patient has no instability when lying down, but, when she attempts either to support herself in an upright position or to sit, she has wild titubation of the trunk and extremities.

Diagnosis

Opsoclonus-myoclonus secondary to neuroblastoma

Ataxia refers to disorders in coordination resulting from errors in timing, rate, and duration of movement. Movement tends to be broken down into its component parts. Cerebellar ataxia is characterized by the following clinical features:

- Wide-based gait with inability to turn on a narrow base
- Vermal lesions: associated with truncal instability
- Hemispheric cerebellar lesions: associated with appendicular ataxia, dysmetria, and dysdiadochokinesia
- Cerebellar tremor: an action-precipitated movement perpendicular to the line of motion
- Reflexes: pendular
- Tone: decreased
- Speech: scanning

DISORDERS OF ATAXIA

Acute

Drugs

These are usually accompanied by nystagmus and/or dysarthria (e.g., Dilantin overdose).

Postinfectious or Infectious (Acute Cerebellar Ataxia)

- Mainly axial ataxia, wide-based gait
- History of recent infection
  - Varicella
  - Coxsackie viruses
  - Echo viruses
- May be associated with vomiting
- Recovery: does occur, but may take weeks to months

Miller Fisher Variety of Guillain-Barré Syndrome

- Cranial neuropathy (bulbar signs)
- Weakness
- Areflexia
- Cerebrospinal fluid: cytoalbumino dissociation
- Treatment: intravenous immunoglobulin

Migraine

For futher discussions of migraine, see Chapter 24. The basilar migraine is associated with acute disorders of ataxia.

Conversion Reaction

- Astasia-abasia
  - Swaying from the waist
  - Wider base does not stabilize gait
- Tone, deep tendon reflexes, coordination: normal

Chronic or Progressive

Developmental

These include structural or congenital defects.

- Basilar impression
- Arnold-Chiari malformation

- Aplasia of the cerebellum
- Dandy-Walker syndrome

Brain Tumors

See Chapter 26 for additional information on ataxia and brain tumors.

- Progressive history, papilledema, and abnormal imaging
- Cerebellar astrocytoma: axial or appendicular ataxia
- Ependymoma: usually axial ataxia
- Medulloblastoma: usually axial ataxia

Paraneoplastic: Neuroblastoma

This is the only known paraneoplastic syndrome seen in children.

- Clinical features
  - Opsoclonus
  - Polymyoclonia
  - Truncal stability
  - Usually a well-differentiated neuroblastoma in the chest
- Evaluation
  - Check urine levels of homovanillic acid (HVA) and vanillylmandelic acid (VMA)
  - Obtain magnetic resonance image of chest and abdomen
- Removal of tumor: symptoms improve
- Intravenous immunoglobulin and steroids: helpful

Encephalopathic (Kinsborne Syndrome)

As with paraneoplastic syndrome, the following are seen:

- Opsoclonus
- Truncal instability
- Polymyoclonia
- Usually 2 to 4 years of age at presentation
- Movements: responsive to corticotropin or prednisone
- Long-term learning disability or decreased intelligence quotient

Genetic (Common Examples)

Recessive

Ataxia Telangiectasia

See Chapter 15 for more information about this condition.

- Gene: 11q
- Seen in 1 in 40,000 births
- Telangiectasia of the conjunctiva, face, chest, and flexor surface of the body
- Progressive truncal ataxia
- Oculomotor apraxias
- Recurrent sinopulmonary infections
- Lymphoreticular neoplasias
- Immunoglobulins A and E (IgA and IgE): absent to diminished

Abetalipoproteinemia (Bassen-Korzweig)

- Ataxia seen in the first decade
- Failure to thrive
- Steatorrhea
- Acanthocytosis
- Retinitis pigmentosa

Friedreich Ataxia

- Triplicate repeat on gene 9q
- Gene: frataxin
- Onset between 2 and 16 years of age
- Ataxia: appendicular and axial
- Dysarthria
- Absent deep tendon reflexes (not invariable)
- Scoliosis
- Pes cavus
- Cardiomyopathy
- Diabetes

Dominant

Spinocerebellar ataxia (Table 31.1) is caused by dominant inheritance.

- At least seven types
- Most are disorders of triplicate repeats that have been mapped to various chromosomes

Clinical Features: Variable

- Optic atrophy
- Retinal changes
- Oculomotor apraxia
- Parkinsonian features
- Progressive ataxia (most prominent feature)

TABLE 31.1 Dominant Forms of Spinocerebellar Ataxia

Type	Chromosome
SCA 1	6q
SCA 2	12q
SCA 3 (Machado-Joseph disease)	14q
SCA 4	4q
SCA 5	11q
SCA 6	19p
SCA 7	3p

Abbreviation: SCA, spinocerebellar ataxia.

RECURRENT ATAXIA

Episodic Ataxia, Type 1

- Mutation of the potassium channel gene: chromosome 12p
- Onset between 5 and 7 years of age
- Duration: minutes to hours
- Responds to acetazolamide

Episodic Ataxia, Type II

- Mutation to chromosome 1q
- Onset: school age to adolescence
- Interictal clumsiness
- Responds to acetazolamide

Metabolic

- Pyruvate decarboxylase deficiency
- Hartnup disease
- Leigh disease
- Ornithine carbamoyltransferase deficiency
- Multiple cocarboxylase deficiency

Paroxysmal Choreoathetosis

See Chapter 32 for further discussion of this condition.

- Kinesiogenic (movement induced)
- Nonkinesiogenic
- Treatment

- Phenytoin
- Carbamazepine
- Acetazolamide
- Artane

Suggested Reading

Benton CS, de Silva R, Rutledge SL, et al. Molecular and clinical studies in SCA-7 define a broad clinical spectrum in infantile phenotype. *Neurology* 1998;51:1081–1086.

Brown DL, Brunt ER, Griggs RC, et al. Identification of two new KCNA1 mutations in episodic ataxia/myokymia families. *Hum Mol Genet* 1995;4:1671–1672.

Brown JR. Examination for ataxia in children. *Mayo Clin Proc* 1971;34:570.

Connolly AM, Dodson WE, Prensky AL, et al. Course and outcome of acute cerebellar ataxia. *Ann Neurol* 1994;35:673–679.

De Michele G, Di Maio L, Filla A, et al. Childhood onset of Friedreich's ataxia: a clinical and genetic study of 36 cases. *Neuropediatrics* 1996; 27:3–7.

Dubourg O, Dürr A, Cancel MS, et al. Analysis of the SCA1 CAG repeat in a large number of families with dominant ataxia: clinical and molecular correlations. *Ann Neurol* 1995;37:176–180.

Durr A, Cossee M, Agid Y, et al. Clinical and genetic abnormalities in patients with Friedreich's ataxia. *N Engl J Med* 1996;335:1169–1175.

Fenichel GM. *Clinical pediatric neurology: a signs and symptoms approach,* 4th ed. Philadelphia: WB Saunders, 2001:231–252.

Frontali M, Spadaro M, Giunti P, et al. Autosomal dominant pure cerebellar ataxia: neurological and genetic study. *Brain* 1992;115:1647–1654.

Geschwind DH, Perlman S, Grody WW, et al. Friedreich's ataxia GAA repeat expansion in patients with recessive or sporadic ataxia. *Neurology* 1997;49:1004–1009.

Gieron-Korthals MA, Westberry KR, Emmanuel PJ. Acute childhood ataxia: 10 year experience. *J Child Neurol* 1994;9:381–384.

Griggs RC, Nutt JG. Episodic ataxias as channelopathies. *Ann Neurol* 1995;37:285–286.

Harding AE. Friedreich's ataxia: a clinical and genetic study of 90 families with an analysis of early diagnostic criteria and intrafamilial clustering of clinical features. *Brain* 1981;104:589–620.

Jacobs BC, Endtz H, van der Meche FG, et al. Serum anti-GQ1b IgG antibodies recognize surface epitopes on *Campylobacter jejuni* from patients with Miller Fisher syndrome. *Ann Neurol* 1995;37:260–264.

Koh PS, Raffensperger JG, Berry S, et al. Long-term outcome in children with opsoclonus-myoclonus and ataxia and coincident neuroblastoma. *J Pediatr* 1994;125:712–716.

Swaiman KF, Zoghbi HY. Cerebellar dysfunction and ataxia in childhood. In: Swaiman KF, Ashwal S, eds. *Pediatric neurology: principles and practice,* 3rd ed. Vol. 2. St. Louis: Mosby, 1999.

Zoghbi HY. The spinocerebellar degenerations. In: Appel SH, ed. *Current neurology.* Vol. 13. St. Louis: Mosby-Year Book, 1993.

Chapter 32

Movement Disorders

Case

An 8-year-old girl presents with a history of quick dance-like movements of the arm that are both distal and proximal. She tends to convert these movements into purposeful activity. This movement has been present for the last 3 or 4 weeks. She now has some difficulty with speech, and she is irritable. The neurologic examination reveals an inability to maintain her tongue protruded and a lack of ability to maintain a steady grip of the examiner's finger. Blood work screening for rheumatic fever and an electrocardiogram are normal.

Diagnosis

A putative diagnosis of Sydenham chorea is made. The patient is placed on haloperidol and penicillin.

Movement disorders are complex disorders of motion. Abnormal movements defy easy editorial description, so they must be visualized to be appreciated. At the time of clinical examination, if the movement disorder is not observed, ask the patient or the patient's family to make a video recording.

Most movements are intermittent and paroxysmal. They may be initiated by movement (Huntington chorea), startle (myoclonus), and stress or emotions (tics). Many abnormalities of movement disappear with sleep, but notable exceptions are seizures, restless leg syndrome, and periodic movements of sleep.

CLINICAL CHARACTERISTICS

- Axial: primarily involves the trunk, with or without titubation (a rhythmic involuntary movement of the head and trunk)
- Appendicular
  - Primarily involves the extremities
  - Proximal
    - Shoulder
    - Pelvic
  - Distal
    - Hand
    - Fingers
    - Legs
    - Bilateral or unilateral
- Opsoclonus
  - Chaotic movements of the eyes
  - Irregular and unpredictable paroxysmal movements

NEUROANATOMY

No well-defined anatomic localization exists for movement disorders, although the extrapyramidal system is commonly implicated. The clinician must remember that normal movement is the result of the complex synthesis of outflow from the pyramidal, extrapyramidal, and cerebellar systems, with each influencing and modulating the effects of the other.

- Extrapyramidal
  - Striatum (i.e., putamen and caudate nucleus)
  - Globus pallidus
  - Substantia nigra
- Cerebellum (see Chapter 31)
  - Vermis (truncal stability)
  - Cerebellar hemisphere (appendicular limb abnormalities of movement and synergy)

CLINICAL DISORDERS

Chorea and Athetosis

These are quick dance-like movements affecting any part of the body in either a stereotyped or rhythmic fashion. In an effort to mask the chorea, a child may attempt to convert an involuntary movement into a purposeful one. Piano-playing movements are commonly used to describe chorea of the hands and fingers.

Chorea can be brought out by asking a child to extend the tongue for 10 to 30 seconds. Inability to maintain the extension of the tongue or a darting in and out of the tongue suggests chorea. The milkmaid sign is the inability to maintain a steady grip of the examiner's finger. The pronator sign is the inability to hold the hands outstretched above the head with the hands facing palms inward. The arms tend to turn into a position of pronation. The shelving sign is hyperextension of the hand when held in a pronated position.

Athetosis is defined as slow writhing movements that primarily involve the distal parts of the extremities. Alternating supination and pronation with movement focused along the long axis of the limb is seen. Heightened emotion or stress may intensify the movement. When the writhing is accompanied by quick movements, it is termed choreoathetosis. Chorea and athetosis are commonly seen in concert (i.e., choreoathetosis). The differential of these conditions is largely the same.

Differential Diagnosis

The differential diagnosis of chorea and/or athetosis or a combination of the two (choreoathetosis) can be quite extensive. The differential should begin with a generic grouping (i.e., congenital, genetic, drugs, infectious, metabolic, neoplastic, vascular, miscellaneous). The following list is not meant to be exhaustive, but it does include the most prominent etiologies.

Etiologies

Congenital

- Kernicterus
- Choreoathetotic cerebral palsy

Hypoxic ischemic

- Ruptured uterus
- Placenta abruptio

Genetic or Degenerative

- Huntington disease: positive family history, absent caudate shadow on computed tomography, triplicate repeats, abnormality found on chromosome 4

- Hallervorden-Spatz disease: positive family history, iron deposits in the basal ganglia, and "tiger eye" on magnetic resonance imaging
- Wilson disease: increased copper levels in the urine, decreased ceruloplasmin levels, Kayser– Fleischer ring, abnormal liver function tests
- Familial paroxysmal choreoathetosis
- Abetalipoproteinemia (Bassen-Korzweig): acanthocytosis, decreased β-lipoproteins, decreased cholesterol levels, retinitis pigmentosa, foul bulky stools

Drugs

- Carbon monoxide
- Heavy metals
- Lithium
- Mercury
- Birth control pills

Infectious

- Poststreptococcal (Sydenham): increased antistreptolysin-O, increased anti-DNAse B, increased antinicotinamide adenine dinucleotide (NAD)ase titers, heart murmur
- Encephalitis

Metabolic

- Hypocalcemia
- Hypoglycemia
- Thyrotoxicosis
- Chorea gravidarum
- Hypoparathyroidism

Neoplastic

Neoplastic etiologies include tumors of the thalamus and basal ganglia.

Collagen–Vascular

- Lupus
- Polyarteritis
- Hyperthyroidism
- Anticardiolipin antibody syndrome

Traumatic

Traumatic causes are the most common etiology of these disorders.

Treatment

Chorea may respond to pharmacotherapy. Commonly used drugs include the following:

- Dopamine receptor blockers
  - Haloperidol
  - Thorazine
- Barbiturates
- Steroids
- Benzodiazepines
  - Diazepam
  - Lorazepam
  - Clonazepam
- Valproic acid
- Penicillin: Sydenham chorea
- Penicillamine: Wilson disease
- Thyroid inhibitors for thyrotoxicosis
- Dopamine for dopamine responsive dystonia (Segawa disease)

Ballismus

Ballismic movements are high amplitude flinging movements of the shoulders or pelvis. These movements are commonly seen in isolation in the child.

Dystonia

Clinical Characteristics

Dystonia is an abnormal attitude of posture that results from co-contraction of the agonist and antagonist muscles. Dystonia may be associated with twisting or turning along the long axis of the body, producing contortions of the body. Dystonia may be associated with the inability to ambulate, stand, or walk. If dystonia involves the bulbar muscles, speech may be severely impaired, resulting in marked dysarthria and unintelligibility.

Spasmodic torticollis, torsion dystonia with equinovarus positioning, and focal dystonia (i.e., writer's cramp, blepharospasm, or spasmodic dystonia) involve selective muscle groups.

Differential Diagnosis of Dystonia

- Drugs: phenothiazines, dopamine receptor blockers
- Hysteria
  - Feigned motor weakness
  - Paroxysmal onset
  - Highly suggestible
  - Improves with reassurance
- Symptomatic
  - Postinfectious
  - Collagen–vascular
  - Traumatic
  - Toxin: carbon monoxide
  - Postinfarction
- Genetic
  - Dystonia musculorum deformans
  - Batten disease
  - Dopa-responsive dystonia (Segawa disease)
  - Paroxysmal choreoathetosis
  - Wilson disease
  - Machado-Joseph disease
  - Huntington disease
  - G_{M1} and G_{M2} gangliosidosis
  - Mitochondrial disease
  - Hallervorden-Spatz disease

Paroxysmal Dystonias

- Paroxysmal dystonic (nonkinesiogenic) choreoathetosis
  - Episodes of dystonia and choreoathetosis
  - Involves the face, arms, trunk, and extremities
  - Lasts minutes to hours
  - May begin at rest
  - Occurs abruptly
  - Suggestively inherited
  - May respond to clonazepam, haloperidol, valproic acid, and acetazolamide
- Paroxysmal kinesiogenic choreoathetosis
  - Briefer than nonkinesiogenic choreoathetosis (less than 2 minutes)
  - May occur up to more than 100 times a day
  - Precipitated by movement, startle, stress, and excitement

- Movements consist of dystonia, choreoathetosis, and ballismus
- May respond to anticonvulsants

- Dopa responsive dystonia (Segawa disease)
  - Autosomal dominant: gene mapped to chromosome 14q
  - Average age of onset: 5 years
  - Diurnal variation with worsening in the evening and improvement in the morning
  - Presents with foot dystonia
  - Features of parkinsonism
  - Responds dramatically to small doses of L-dopa

Suggested Reading

Aron AM, Freeman JM, Carter S. The natural history of Sydenham's chorea. *Am J Med* 1965;38:83–95.

Berrios X, Quesney F, Morales A, et al. Are all recurrences of "pure" Sydenham chorea true recurrences of acute rheumatic fever? *J Pediatr* 1985;107:867–872.

Cardoso F, Eduardo C, Silva AP, Mota C. Chorea in fifty consecutive patients with rheumatic fever. *Mov Disord* 1997;12:701–703.

Chase TN, Friedhoff AJ, Cohen DJ, eds. Tourette syndrome: genetics, neurobiology, and treatment. *Adv Neurol* 1992;58.

Deonna T. DOPA-sensitive progressive dystonia of childhood with fluctuations of symptoms: Segawa's syndrome and possible variants. Results of a collaborative study of the European Federation of Child Neurology Societies (EFCNS). *Neuropediatrics* 1986;17:81–85.

Erickson GR, Chun RW. Acquired paroxysmal movement disorders. *Pediatr Neurol* 1987;3:226–229.

Goodenough DJ, Fariello RG, Annis BL, Chun RW. Familial and acquired paroxysmal dyskinesias. *Arch Neurol* 1978;35:827–831.

Nygaard TG, Marsden CD, Fahn S. Dopa-responsive dystonia: long-term treatment response and prognosis. *Neurology* 1991;41:174–181.

Robinson RO, Thornett CE. Benign hereditary chorea: response to steroids. *Dev Med Child Neurol* 1985;27:814–816.

Schwartz A, Hennerici M, Wegener OH. Delayed choreoathetosis following acute carbon monoxide poisoning. *Neurology* 1985;35:98—99.

Stevens H. Paroxysmal choreoathetosis. *Arch Neurol* 1966;14:415–420.

Swedo SE, Leonard HL, Garvey M, et al. Pediatric autoimmune neuropsychiatric disorders associated with streptococcal infections: clinical description of the first 50 cases. *Am J Psychiatry* 1998;155:264–271.

Tadzynski LA, Ryan ME. Diagnosis of rheumatic fever. A guide to the criteria and manifestations. *Postgrad Med* 1986;79:295–300.

Chapter 33

Other Movement Disorders: Myoclonus, Tics, and Tremors

Case

A 9-year-old boy is brought to the office with a history of vocal and motor tics that have been occurring for the past year. The motor tics are primarily oral-buccal in nature, affecting the shoulders and face. The mother is being treated for an obsessive-compulsive disorder. An associated history of obsessive-compulsive disorder and attention deficit disorder is present. The child is doing poorly in school, and he has poor social interrelations.

Diagnosis

Tourette syndrome

MYOCLONUS

Myoclonus is defined as rapid jerking of a muscle or group of muscles, usually with displacement of a joint. Myoclonus can be focal or generalized, rhythmic or arrhythmic, and spontaneous, or accentuated by movement. Most myoclonus is attenuated by sleep, although benign sleep myoclonus is well known in all age groups. Myoclonus activated by movement is labeled as action myoclonus. Myoclonus brought out by sensory stimulation is called reflex sensitive myoclonus.

Opsoclonus is rapid, usually conjugate, chaotic, dancing eye movements. The movements are rarely dysconjugate, and, on occasion, they are associated with oscillopsia—the sensation of visual movement when the eyes move from one position to another.

Classification

- Epileptic or nonepileptic
- Physiologic
  - Benign
  - Sleep, exercise, or stress induced
- Pathologic
  - Generalized
  - Subcortical
  - Brainstem
  - Spinal cord
- Progressive or nonprogressive
- Negative tone (i.e., asterixis—the loss of tone): initiate by asking the patient to hold the hands outstretched. A paroxysmal loss of the extensor tone at the wrist may be seen.

Clinical Entities

- Epilepsy: juvenile myoclonic epilepsy, infantile spasms
- Hypoxic-ischemic state
- Basal ganglia disorders
  - Huntington disease
  - Hallervorden-Spatz disease
  - Wilson disease
- Drug induced
  - Valproic acid
  - Carbamazepine
  - Tricyclics
- Storage disease
- Metabolic encephalopathy: asterixis seen primarily with these conditions
  - Liver failure
  - Renal failure
  - Electrolyte imbalance
- Infectious
  - Encephalitis
  - Subacute sclerosing panencephalitis (SSPE)
  - Parainfectious encephalopathy

TICS

Tics are sudden stereotypic movements that can be either motor or vocal. They are involuntary, and, with effort, they can be suppressed. Unlike chorea, they are readily reproducible by the patient and the observer.

Clinical Characteristics

- Increase with stress
- Usually not seen in sleep
- Usually proximal or oral buccal
- Begin in the last half of the first decade of life; may be lifelong

Types

- Simple: eye blinking, shoulder shrugs, arm and leg shrugs
- Complex: rubbing, bruxism, jumping, skipping, hopping, echopraxia
- Vocal: can be simple or complex, such as grunting, snorting, barking or neologisms, panting, whistling, coprolalia, and incomprehensible noises

TREMOR

Tremors are rhythmic, oscillating movements with a predictable speed, amplitude, and force. They may be slow or rapid.

Familial

- Usually autosomal dominant
- Involves hands and may spread proximally; the "no" tremor of head and chin is common
- Increase with volition and decrease with sleep
- Relieved by beta-blockers and ethanol

Postural Tremor

This tremor is present when the arms are extended. The frequency of the tremor may change over time; it is suppressed by adrenergic blockers. These tremors are increased by fatigue and anxiety, hyperthyroidism, and epinephrine agonists.

Spasmus Nutans

Spasmus nutans is horizontal bobbing (the "no" tremor) of the head; it is associated with nystagmus of either both or one eye.

- Age at onset: 3 months to 1 year
- Resolves by 2 to 4 years of age
- Must exclude chiasmatic gliomas

TOURETTE SYNDROME

Tics

Tourette syndrome is characterized by a vocal or motor tic that is present for more than 1 year.

Associated Features

- Obsessive-compulsive disorder
- Attention deficit disorder
- Familial association (look for isolated obsessive-compulsive disorder or attention deficit hyperactivity disorder without tics in families)

Treatment

- Dopamine receptor blockers
- Clonidine
- Pimozide
- Selective serotonin reuptake inhibitors
- Counseling

Suggested Reading

Bienfang DC. Opsoclonus in infancy. *Arch Ophthalmol* 1974;91:203–205.

Busenbark K, Barnes P, Lyons K, et al. Accuracy of reported family histories of essential tremor. *Neurology* 1996;47:264–265.

Cohen DJ, Bruun RD, Leckman JF, eds. *Tourette's syndrome and tic disorders.* New York: John Wiley & Sons, 1988.

Golden GS. Tourette syndrome: recent advances. *Pediatr Neurol* 1986;2: 189–192.

Shapiro E, Shapiro AK. Semiology, nosology, and criteria for tic disorders. *Rev Neurol (Paris)* 1986;142:824–832.

Swaiman KF. Hallervorden-Spatz syndrome and brain iron metabolism. *Arch Neurol* 1991;48:1285–1293.

Swaiman KF. Myoclonus. *Neurol Clin* 1985;3:197–208.

Swanson PO, Luttrell CM, Magladery JW. Myoclonus: a report of 67 cases and review of the literature. *Medicine* 1962;41:339.

Warrier RP, Kini R, Besser A, et al. Opsomyoclonus and neuroblastoma. *Clin Pediatr (Phila)* 1985;24:32–34.

Chapter 34

Pervasive Developmental Disorders

Case

A 6-year-old child with a history of poor social interaction, failure to make eye contact, and failure to develop peer relationships appropriate to his developmental level is seen. The child also has difficulty with the spoken language, and he has demonstrated repetitive and stereotypic patterns of behavior, interests, and activities.

Diagnosis

Pervasive developmental disorder, autistic type

The term pervasive developmental disorder (PDD) embraces a spectrum of behavioral syndromes that are characterized by abnormalities in socialization, communication, and personality integration. This spectrum of disease, although considered to have a genetic basis, has no known etiologic cause. Rather, PDD consists of a variety of presentations, and multifactorial in origin. The observation that several genetic abnormalities may have a phenotype suggestive of PDD has given credence to a putative genetic etiology.

The following five conditions are listed in the *Diagnostic and Statistical Manual of Mental Disorders,* 4th edition, text revision (DSM-IV-TR), as PDDs: (a) classic autism; (b) Rett syndrome; (c) disintegrative disorder; (d) Asperger syndrome; and (e) PDD, not otherwise classified. All five syndromes begin in childhood usually before

2 or 3 years of age. Although some patients may improve, few rarely fully recover. The epidemiology is unclear. The incidence of PDD may be increasing to as high as 1.4 per 100,000 individuals under 10 years of age, and it is more common in boys than it is in girls. Up to 30% will have electroencephalographic abnormalities and even frank seizures.

AUTISM

Etiology

- Genetic
  - Concordance in twins: 60% to 70%
  - Less than 10% recurrence in sibships
- Disease associations
  - Fragile X
  - Angelman syndrome
  - Landau-Kleffner syndrome (acquired epileptic aphasia)
  - Tuberous sclerosis
  - May be seen following encephalitis or trauma
  - PANDAS (pediatric autoimmune neuropsychiatric disorder associated with streptococcus)
- Nonspecific pathology
  - Large head: may or may not be present
  - Developmental abnormalities in the cerebellum
  - Suggestive involvement of the dopaminergic and serotonergic neurotransmitter systems

Symptomatology

- Six of the 12 descriptors from the DSM-IV (Table 34.1), including two involving sociability and one each in language and communication
- Nonverbal
- No interest in environmental happenings
- Stereotypies, such as flapping of the hands, rocking, whirling, and pacing
- Echolalia or echopraxia
- Failure to point to indicate needs
- Hyperreaction and hyporeaction to sensory stimuli
- Failure to respond to environmental clues

TABLE 34.1 Diagnostic and Statistical Manual of Mental Disorders, 4th edition, Diagnostic Criteria for Autistic Disorder

A. A total of six (or more) items from 1, 2, and 3, with at least two items from 1 and one each from 2 and 3.
   1. Qualitative impairment in social interaction, as manifested by at least two of the following:
      a. Marked impairment in the use of multiple nonverbal behaviors, such as eye-to-eye gaze, facial expression, body postures, and gestures to regulate social interaction.
      b. Failure to develop peer relationships appropriate to developmental level.
      c. A lack of spontaneous seeking to share enjoyment, interests, or achievements with other people (e.g., by a lack of showing, bringing, or pointing out objects of interest).
      d. Lack of social or emotional reciprocity.
   2. Qualitative impairment in communication as manifested by at least one of the following:
      a. Delay in, or total lack of, the development of spoken language (not accompanied by attempts to compensate through alternative modes of communication, such as gestures or mime).
      b. In individuals with adequate speech, marked impairment in the ability to initiate or sustain a conversation with others.
      c. Stereotyped and repetitive use of language or idiosyncratic language.
      d. Lack of varied, spontaneous make believe play or social imitative play appropriate to developmental level.
   3. Restricted repetitive and stereotyped patterns of behavior, interests, and activities, as manifested by at least one of the following:
      a. Encompassing preoccupation with one or more stereotyped and restricted patterns of interest that is abnormal either in intensity or focus.
      b. Apparently inflexible adherence to specific, nonfunctional routines or rituals.
      c. Stereotyped and repetitive motor mannerisms (e.g., hand or finger flapping or twisting or complex whole-body movements).
      d. Persistent preoccupation with parts of objects.

B. Delays or abnormal functioning in at least one of the following areas, with onset before the age of 3: (a) social interaction, (b) language as used in social communication, or (c) symbolic or imaginative play.

C. The disturbance is not better accounted by Rett disorder or childhood disintegrative disorder.

From the American Psychiatric Association. *Diagnostic and statistical manual of mental disorders,* 4th ed. Washington, D.C.: American Psychiatric Press, 1994, with permission.

Language Abnormalities

- Pragmatics: failure to develop normal nonverbal aspects of communication (i.e., pointing, gestures, and imitation)
- Semantic: failure to understand meanings of words and phrases and abnormal syntax
- Phonology: abnormal rhythm and flow of language (i.e., high-pitched sounds, rising inflection in speech, and metallic quality to speech)

Cognition

- The intelligence quotient may be normal.
- Most fall into the educable mentally retarded (EMR) range.
- Intellectual performance is uneven.
- The child tends to have intact spatial-visual abilities with a disability in verbal tasks.

RETT SYNDROME

- Progressive, with loss of ambulation, seizures, and sleep disturbances
- Almost exclusively affects girls unlike classic autism
- Genetic defect: the *MECP2* gene on the X chromosome
- Plateau of head circumference; eventually diagnosed as microcephalic
- Associated seizures
- Stereotypies, such as hand flapping and wringing of the hands
- Late development of long tract signs
- Hypoventilation and hyperventilation: may occur late in the course of the disease

DISINTEGRATIVE DISORDER

- Rarest syndrome
- Catastrophic regression in language, sociability, and cognition
- Usually occurs in preschool years
- Electroencephalogram: suggests acquired epileptic aphasia

ASPERGER SYNDROME

- Normal expressive language

- Intelligence quotient: usually normal or in the highly educable range
- Described as "nerds" (i.e., intellectual, little professor), appear to have deep and profound interests
- Social ineptitude
- Abnormal or complete absence of peer relationships
- Rigid
- Unaware of how others perceive them

PERVASIVE DEVELOPMENTAL DISORDER, NOT OTHERWISE SPECIFIED

Definition

This diagnosis is reserved for those who have abnormalities of sociability, cognition, and language and who do not fall easily into the other DSM-IV categories. This may be less severe than other syndromes.

Treatment

- Education
  - Small classes
  - Language and speech therapy
  - Structured environment
  - Parental education
  - Behavioral management
- Pharmacotherapy (largely a matter of trial and error)
  - Serotonin uptake inhibitors
  - α-Adrenergic agonists
  - β-Adrenergic inhibitors
  - Anxiolytic
  - Stimulants
  - Antidepressants
  - Anticonvulsants
  - Hypnotics

Suggested Reading

American Psychiatric Association. *Diagnostic and statistical manual of mental disorders,* 4th ed. Text revision. Washington, D.C.: American Psychiatric Association, 2000.

Filipek PA, Accardo PJ, Ashwal S, et al. Practice parameter: screening and diagnosis of autism. Report of the Quality Standards Committee of the American Academy of Neurology and the Child Neurology Society. *Neurology* 2000;55:468–479.

Filipek PA, Accardo PJ, Baranek GT, et al. The screening and diagnosis of autistic spectrum disorders. *J Autism Dev Disord* 1999;29:439–484.

Naidu S. Rett syndrome: a disorder affecting early brain growth. *Ann Neurol* 2001;42:3–10.

Rodier PM. The early origins of autism. *Sci Am* 2000;282:56–63.

Chapter 35

Attention Deficit Hyperactivity Disorder

Case

A 6-year-old child is referred by the school because of poor performance. The child is highly distractible, inattentive, impulsive, and hyperactive. His intelligence quotient is normal, but his failure to stay on task has interfered with his performance. The father had similar problems as a child.

Diagnosis

Attention deficit hyperactivity disorder

Attention deficit disorders are the most common behavioral disorders of childhood. Prevalence rates vary, but they are reported to be between 2% and 15% in the general population. This syndrome occurs cross-culturally in children and adolescents. It may be found in families and may persist into adulthood. The male-to-female ratio is 2 to 1.

CLINICAL FEATURES: THREE CARDINAL FEATURES

- Inattention
- Impulsivity
- Hyperactivity

ASSOCIATED PROBLEMS

- Tourette syndrome

- Learning disabilities
- Thyroid disorders
- Psychiatric problems
  - Dysfunctional families
  - Conduct disorder
  - Bipolar disorder
- May develop after head trauma, meningitis, encephalitis, radiation, and chemotherapy to the central nervous sytem or after any other abnormality associated with damage to the central nervous system

EVALUATION

- Biologic or radiologic markers that help to establish the diagnosis: none
- Diagnosis: made on clinical grounds

MULTIMODAL TREATMENT

- Family therapy
- Behavioral modification techniques: used at home and in the school setting
- Pharmacotherapy: used as an adjunct to other treatments
  - Stimulants (see Appendix VIII)
    - Ritalin
    - Adderall
    - Concerta
    - Pemoline
    - *Side effects:* decreased appetite, sleep disturbances, mood disorders, tics (rare), and decreases in growth (rare)
  - Antidepressants
    - Tricyclics (imipramine, nortriptyline)
    - Wellbutrin
    - Effexor
    - Prozac
    - *Side effects:* constipation, dry mouth, cardiac conduction defects, rash, and insomnia
  - Antihypertensives
    - Clonidine
    - *Side effects:* sedation, decreased blood pressure, confusion, dry mouth, somnolence, and headache

Suggested Reading

American Psychiatry Association. *Diagnostic and statistical manual of mental disorders,* 4th ed. Text revision. Washington, D.C.: American Psychiatric Association, 2000.

Lambert NM, Sandoval J. The prevalence of learning disabilities in a sample of children considered hyperactive. *J Abnorm Child Psychol* 1980;8:33–50.

Wasserman RC, Kelleher KJ, Bocian A, et al. Identification of attentional and hyperactivity problems in primary care: a report from pediatric research in office settings and the ambulatory sentinel practice network. *Pediatrics* 1999;103:E38.

Wolraich ML, Hannah JN, Pinnock JY, et al. Comparison of diagnostic criteria for attention-deficit hyperactivity disorder in a county-wide sample. *J Am Acad Child Adolesc Psychiatry* 1996;35:319–324.

Zametkin A, Rapoport JL. The neurobiology of attention deficit disorder with hyperactivity: where have we come in 50 years? *J Am Acad Child Adolesc Psychiatry* 1987;26:676–686.

Chapter 36

Vertigo

Case

A 2-year-old child suddenly tells his mother that he is unsteady and is going to fall. He is fully alert but is obviously frightened and ataxic. The mother notes jerking movements of his eyes. The episode, which lasts 5 minutes, is followed by complete recovery.

Diagnosis

Benign paroxysmal vertigo

Vertigo is an illusion of rotation of either the subject or the environment. Vertigo must be distinguished from light-headedness.

HISTORY

Duration

- Episodes lasting seconds: benign positional vertigo
- Episodes lasting minutes: migraine, vertebrobasilar insufficiency (transient ischemic attack), and vestibulogenic epilepsy
- Episodes lasting hours: Ménière syndrome
- Episodes lasting days: vestibular neuritis, trauma, or infarction labyrinth

Tempo

- Abrupt: trauma, vascular occlusion
- Gradual (hours to days): vestibular neuritis (viral)

Associated Symptoms and Location

- Nausea, vomiting, diaphoresis, pallor: typically associated with peripheral vestibular dysfunction (nystagmus toward the affected side is often present)
- Hearing loss (abrupt), tinnitus, pressure, or pain in ear: lesion of the labyrinth or eighth nerve (inner ear)
- Hearing loss, tinnitus, facial weakness (ipsilateral): lesion of the internal auditory canal
- Ipsilateral facial weakness, facial numbness, limb ataxia, hearing loss (progressive), tinnitus: lesion in the cerebellar pontine angle
- Cranial nerves, ataxia, long tract signs, drop attacks, hearing intact: lesion in the brainstem
- Ataxia with intact hearing: lesion in the cerebellum
- Abnormal taste, odors, confusion, altered consciousness: partial complex seizures, indicating a lesion of the temporal lobe

Past History

- Recent viral infection (vestibular neuritis)
- Head injury (labyrinthine trauma)
- Diabetes

Birth History

- Congenital infections (may lead to recurrent episodes of vertigo), including toxoplasmosis, cytomegalovirus, herpes, bacterial or viral meningitis, and acquired immunodeficiency syndrome
- Hyperbilirubinemia
- Perinatal asphyxia
- Drug exposure (see below)

Drug History

- Ototoxic drugs (aminoglycosides)
- Antihypertensives (presyncopal light-headedness)
- Anticoagulants: hemorrhage in the inner ear
- Phenytoin (ataxia)
- Alcohol: positional vertigo
- Sedatives: disorientation rather than vertigo

Family History

- Ménière syndrome
- Migraine
- Neurofibromatosis, type 2 (acoustic neuromas)
- Spinocerebellar degeneration
- von Hippel-Lindau disease

BEDSIDE TEST FOR VESTIBULAR DYSFUNCTION: DIX-HALLPIKE MANEUVER

Positional testing is performed with the patient being brought from the sitting to the supine position with the head hanging 45 degrees below the horizontal. Then head is turned once to the right and once to the left to induce paroxysmal positional nystagmus or vertigo or both.

Peripheral Vestibular Syndromes

Spontaneous nystagmus occurs away from the affected labyrinth. Past pointing and falling toward the affected side is present. Caloric testing shows ipsilateral canal paresis with absent nystagmus on stimulation of the affected ear or directional preponderance to the contralateral side.

Central Vestibular Syndromes

Dix-Hallpike elicits nystagmus in all directions. Caloric testing does not indicate canal paresis, but directional preponderance may be present. The hearing is intact.

DIFFERENTIAL DIAGNOSIS

Acute Vertigo with Hearing Loss

- Labyrinthitis
  - History of infection
  - Autonomic symptoms: present
  - Unstable gait
  - Spontaneous fast nystagmus toward the normal ear
  - Most comfortable lying on the unaffected side
  - Duration: days

- Ménière disease (uncommon in children)
  - Vertigo
  - Fluctuating hearing loss
  - Pressure in the ear
  - Tinnitus
- Temporal bone fracture
- Perilymphatic fistula (trauma)
- Vascular occlusion

Paroxysmal Vertigo Without Hearing Loss

- Benign paroxysmal vertigo (recurrent)
  - Age at onset: 16 months to 2 years; gone by 4 years of age
  - Nystagmus: usually present
  - Vomiting: uncommon
  - No loss of consciousness
  - Migraine variant
  - Obtain electroencephalogram to exclude seizure disorder
  - Electronystagmography (ENG): hypoactive labyrinth
- Head trauma leading to labyrinthine concussion
  - Trauma to the parietooccipital or the temporoparietal region
  - Vertigo, falling toward the affected side
  - Nausea and vomiting
  - Paroxysmal positional nystagmus (Dix-Hallpike)
  - ENG: decreased function of the labyrinth
  - Duration: 3 to 6 weeks
- Basilar migraine (see Chapter 24 for futher discussion)
- Vertiginous epilepsy: form of partial complex seizures
- Vestibular neuronitis
  - Follows respiratory infection
  - Acute onset of vertigo
  - Nausea, vomiting, and instability
  - May recur
  - ENG: indicates positional nystagmus
  - Treatment: antihistamines, meclizine
- Whiplash injury
  - May be due to cervical muscle spasm that causes impaired vertebrobasilar circulation
  - Symptoms subside in a few months
  - ENG: shows positional nystagmus
  - Treatment: diazepam can be helpful

Chronic Vertigo With Hearing Loss Either With or Without Neurologic Abnormalities

- Acoustic neuroma
- Cerebellopontine angle tumor
- Posterior fossa tumor
- Drug induced
- Cholesteatoma
- Cerebrovascular accident
- Friedrich ataxia
- Refsum disease

Chronic Vertigo Without Hearing Loss or Neurologic Abnormalities

- Hematologic: sickle cell anemia
- Metabolic: diabetes mellitus
- Vertebrobasilar insufficiency
- Ototoxic drugs: often have hearing loss
- Psychosomatic

LIGHT-HEADEDNESS: A FEELING OF IMPENDING SYNCOPE

Etiologies

- Orthostatic hypotension
  - Neurocardiogenic syncope: may or may not be present
  - Postural orthostatic tachycardia syndrome: may or may not be present
- Vasovagal attack
- Hyperventilation
- Decreased cardiac output
  - Arrhythmia
  - Vascular disease
  - Heart failure
- Psychologic dizziness: anxiety attacks or panic attacks
  - Shortness of breath
  - Increased heart rate
  - Diaphoresis
  - Tingling
  - Trembling and shaking
  - Fear of dying

Suggested Reading

Eviatar L. Vertigo. In: Swaiman KF, Ashwal S, eds. *Pediatric neurology: principles & practice,* 3rd ed. Vol. 1. St. Louis: Mosby-Year Book, 1999.

Eviatar L, Eviatar A. Vertigo in children: differential diagnosis and treatment. *Pediatrics* 1977;59:833—838.

Lanzi G, Balottin U, Fazzi E, et al. Benign paroxysmal vertigo of childhood: a long-term follow-up. *Cephalalgia* 1994;14:458–460.

Schick B, Brors D, Koch O, et al. Magnetic resonance imaging in patients with sudden hearing loss, tinnitus and vertigo. *Otol Neurotol* 2001; 22:808–812.

Weisleder P, Fife TD. Dizziness and headache: a common association in children and adolescents. *J Child Neurol* 2001;16:727–730.

Chapter 37

Lumbar Puncture and Cerebrospinal Fluid Examination

INDICATIONS

- Lumbar puncture (LP) is performed whenever infection is suspected. The exception to this is that LP should not be performed if a brain abscess or another space-occupying lesion is suspected.
- LP is used to diagnose subarachnoid hemorrhage when the neuroimaging is negative.
- LP is conducted to obtain diagnostic information.
  - Gamma globulin and oligoclonal banding in multiple sclerosis
  - Metabolic studies (e.g., hyperglycinemia)
- LP is obtained to measure spinal fluid pressure.
  - Check for increased pressure in suspected pseudotumor cerebri
  - Check for low pressure in spontaneous intracranial hypotension headache
  - Used occasionally to measure pressure in patients with hydrocephalus
- LP is used for cytology to diagnose leptomeningeal disease.
- LP is used therapeutically in the following ways:
  - Installation of chemotherapeutic agents (e.g., methotrexate)
  - Insertion of antibiotics
  - Removal of spinal fluid as treatment for benign increased intracranial pressure

CONTRAINDICATIONS

- When infection is present at the site of the LP
- When the patient has a bleeding disorder or thrombocytopenia

- When suspicion of the presence of a mass lesion, such as blood, pus, or tumor
- Spinal block: relative contraindication. Neuroimaging should be done before conducting the LP.
- Presence of papilledema: contraindicated, except to diagnose pseudotumor cerebri

COMPLICATIONS

- LP headache
  - Occurs in 10% to 30% of patients
  - Exacerbated by sitting or standing
  - Relieved by lying flat
  - Occurs 1 to 3 days after LP; may last from several days to several weeks
  - Believed to be due to continuous leakage of cerebrospinal fluid through a dural tear at the site of the spinal tap
  - Treatment
    - Complete bed rest for 24 hours
    - Abdominal binder
    - Forced fluids
    - Occasionally use blood patch, but risk of infection
  - Prevention: use a 22-gauge needle and a single effort rather than multiple efforts to minimize the occurrence of post-spinal fluid headache
- Unexpected increased opening pressure
  - In the presence of increased intracranial pressure, minimal amounts of fluid should be removed. The patient should be watched carefully over the following hours for signs of deterioration. Neurosurgical consultation may be necessary.
  - Patients with meningitis may have markedly elevated pressures, but this is usually not a problem because the pressure is distributed equally throughout the nervous system. This finding is not associated with the movement of tissue from an area of high resistance to low resistance and subsequent herniation.
  - Hypercarbia, water intoxication, and hypertensive encephalopathy are causes of increased intracranial pressure.
  - Spinal block is suggested by findings of low to absent spinal fluid pressures, xanthochromia, and a high protein level.

In these situations, neurosurgical consultation is required to rule out the presence of compressive disease of the spinal cord.

METHODOLOGY

- The puncture is carried out in the midline between the L-3 and L-4 interspace located at the level of the iliac crest.
- The bevel of the needle is inserted parallel to the long axis of the spine.
- Manometric studies are best obtained using a 20-gauge needle.
- Opening and closing pressures should be recorded.
- Coughing or pressure on the abdomen should cause an increased rise in spinal fluid in the manometer. This indicates free flow in the subarachnoid space.
- Proper positioning is crucial for a successful spinal tap. The patient is placed in the lateral decubitus position. The needle is inserted parallel to the bed and is angled toward the patient's umbilicus. With experience, the clinician can recognize a familiar "pop" as the needle enters the subarachnoid space.
- If the LP is unobtainable in the lateral decubitus, sitting the patient up increases the spinal fluid pressure by hydrostatic mechanisms. This increases the size of the subarachnoid space, making entering the subarachnoid space easier.

EXAMINATION OF THE SPINAL FLUID

- Collect four tubes of spinal fluid
  - First tube: cell count
  - Second tube: chemistries
  - Third tube: bacteriologic studies
  - Fourth tube: save for future use
- Suspected traumatic tap
  - Count cells in first and second tubes.
  - Fluid should be spun down to determine if xanthochromia is present. The absence of xanthochromia in the presence of red cells suggests a traumatic tap.
- Compare spinal fluid to water
  - A cerebrospinal fluid protein level greater than 100 mg may cause the spinal fluid to look faintly xanthochromic.

- ◆ At least 200 to 300 white cells are usually needed to cause cloudiness of the spinal fluid.
- ◆ Xanthochromia is seen with hyperbilirubinemia and subarachnoid blood.
- ◆ The spinal fluid should be examined for cells within 1 hour of the LP to eliminate the potential for hemolysis.
- ◆ The protein content is increased by approximately 1 mg per dL by 700 to 1,000 red blood cells.
- ◆ One white cell is found for every 700 red blood cells.

- ■ Interpretation
  - ◆ Glucose: increased glucose levels are usually insignificant, reflecting only systemic hyperglycemia. Spinal fluid sugar lags behind blood glucose levels by several hours. Normal spinal fluid level is approximately two-thirds that of blood glucose.
    - Bacterial, tuberculous, and fungal meningitis: decreased glucose levels. Decreased glucose is also seen in carcinomatous meningitis and nontuberculous granulomatous processes, such as sarcoidosis.
    - Bacterial infection: the spinal fluid sugar is invariably below 20 mg %, independent of systemic glucose.
  - ◆ Protein: increased protein levels are seen in multiple neurologic diseases; usually reflect either disruption of the blood–brain barrier or irritation of the ependymal or meningeal surfaces of the brain.
    - Normal spinal fluid protein: less than 45 mg %.
    - Infants born prematurely and newborns: spinal fluid protein, for the first month of life, may be as high as 100 to 150 mg per dL.
- ■ Common processes associated with increased spinal fluid protein
  - ◆ Diabetes causes protein elevations up to 150 mg per mL.
  - ◆ Brain tumors may increase the protein level, specifically when the tumor is near an ependymal surface or the meninges.
  - ◆ Spinal cord tumors in the presence of a block may have a protein concentration over 1 g per dL.
  - ◆ Demyelinating disease is associated with mild increases in protein.
  - ◆ Purulent meningitis, viral meningitis, and encephalitis are all associated with increased protein concentrations.

- Carcinomatous meningitis and leptomeningeal disease are associated with significant increases in spinal fluid protein.
- Guillain-Barré syndrome is characteristically associated with increased protein levels in the absence of cells.

■ Pleocytosis
- Polymorphonuclear leukocytes in the spinal fluid should always suggest bacterial infection.
- "Polys" are not native to the nervous system; they are always blood-borne.
- Lymphocytes may suggest a chronic inflammatory process. Five to six mononuclear cells are considered normal.
- White blood cells may be seen with subarachnoid hemorrhage and intracranial bleeding.
- Eosinophils suggest a parasitic reaction.
- Carcinomatous meningitis may be accompanied by fewer than 100 cells in the spinal fluid. T-cell and B-cell markers should be checked if the spinal fluid protein level is elevated and lymphomatous meningitis is suspected.
- Three serial taps should be done to exclude leptomeningeal disease.

■ Cerebrospinal fluid pressure
- The cerebrospinal fluid pressure is usually less than 200 mm H_2O with the patient lying down and legs extended.
- In the sitting position, the pressure will normally rise to the level of the ventricular system because no valves are present in the spinal fluid; this depends on the height of the individual.
- Elevated pressure can be seen in bacterial, fungal, and viral meningitis and with intracranial mass lesions.
- Pressure may be elevated in intracranial bleeding.
- Spinal fluid pressure *rarely* may be elevated in cases of polyneuritis or Guillain-Barré syndrome.
- An unexplained elevation of pressure can be caused by heart failure, chronic obstructive pulmonary disease, hypercapnia, pericardial effusion, and jugular venous obstruction.
- Pseudotumor cerebri is associated with pressures as high as 400 to 600 mm H_2O (see Chapter 28).
- Posturally dependent headaches are associated with low spinal fluid pressure.

Suggested Reading

Ahmed A, Hickey SM, Ehrett S, et al. Cerebrospinal fluid values in the term neonate. *Pediatr Infect Dis J* 1996;15:298–303.

Bonadio WA, Smith DS, Metrou M, Dewitz B. Estimating lumbar-puncture depth in children. *N Engl J Med* 1988;319:952–953.

Duffy GP. Lumbar puncture in the presence of raised intracranial pressure. *BMJ* 1969;1:407–409.

Ellis RW 3rd, Strauss LC, Wiley JM, et al. A simple method of estimating cerebrospinal fluid pressure during lumbar puncture. *Pediatrics* 1992; 89:895–897.

Fishman RA. *Cerebrospinal fluid in diseases of the nervous system,* 2nd ed. Philadelphia: WB Saunders, 1992.

Portnoy JM, Olson LC. Normal cerebrospinal fluid values in children: another look. *Pediatrics* 1985;75:484–487.

Appendix I

Key Developmental Milestones

FIRST 4 WEEKS

- Clears airway
- Legs flexed in prone position
- Active stepping and placing
- Vigorous Moro reflex
- Visually attentive

SKILLS AT 4 WEEKS

- Raises head in prone position
- Hands open 50% of time
- Legs extended in prone position
- Spontaneous smile

SKILLS AT 8 WEEKS

- Raises head and chest in prone position
- Follows object
- Can easily flex legs when held in vertical position with pressure applied over pelvis
- Social smile

SKILLS AT 12 WEEKS

- Hands open most of the time
- Follows with eyes through 180 degrees

- Regards face
- Hands come to midline

SKILLS AT 16 WEEKS

- Legs extended
- Chest raised, begins to extend chest in prone position
- Axial control developing
- Beginning to bear weight
- Spontaneous laughter
- Reaches and grabs

SKILLS AT 28 WEEKS

- Rolls over
- Sits in "C" position
- Axial tone increasing
- Bounces on feet, bears weight
- Palmar grasp
- Transfers objects, rakes objects
- Babbling

SKILLS AT 40 WEEKS

- Sits unsupported
- Cruises along furniture
- Inferior prehension
- Picks up small objects
- Waves bye-bye, peekaboo
- Points to parts of face
- Socially interactive

SKILLS AT 1 YEAR

- Knows family members
- Walks either alone or holding on to one hand
- Developing pincer grasp, picks up small objects
- Watches self in mirror
- Has a 3-word to 10-word vocabulary

SKILLS AT 15 MONTHS

- Walks by self
- Cruises up and down stairs
- Inserts pellet in bottle, makes a tower of three
- Points at objects
- Stranger anxiety

SKILLS AT 18 MONTHS

- Runs awkwardly
- May have 10-word to 20-word vocabulary
- Identifies parts of the body
- Plays simple ball games
- Responds enthusiastically to family members
- Puts food in mouth

SKILLS AT 2 YEARS

- Increased dexterity
- Runs well, climbs stairs
- Scribbles
- Puts three words together, vocabulary increasing
- Increasing demands and desires
- Stranger anxiety

SKILLS AT 3 YEARS

- Counts to 10 and above
- Rides tricycle with training wheels
- Undresses self, helps dress self
- Speaks in full sentences
- Socially interactive
- Knows colors
- Climbs stairs
- Can draw a circle

SKILLS AT 4 YEARS

- Beginning toilet training
- Parallel play

- Hops and skips
- Speaks in full complex sentences
- Syntax developing
- Can draw a cross
- Draws head with arms and legs attached to head
- Counts to 10 and above
- Social play with others
- Cuts along a line
- Increased motor skills
- Uses scissors

SKILLS AT 5 YEARS

- Rides bike
- Tells story
- Prints name
- Learning the alphabet
- Beginning to read
- Dresses and undresses
- Responds readily to routine assignments of tasks
- Readily participates in group activities
- Draws a triangle
- Knows phone number and address

Appendix II

Newborn Maturity Rating and Classification

DUBOWITZ AND BALLARD EXAMINATION FOR GESTATIONAL AGE

Neuromuscular Maturity

See Fig. II.1.

Posture

With the infant supine and quiet, score as follows:

- Arms and legs extended = 0
- Slight or moderate flexion of the hips and knees = 1
- Moderate to strong flexion of the hips and knees = 2
- Legs flexed and abducted, arms slightly flexed = 3
- Full flexion of the arms and legs = 4

Square Window

Flex the hand at the wrist. Exert sufficient pressure to get as much flexion as possible. The angle between the hypothenar eminence and the anterior aspect of the forearm is measured and scored as follows:

- More than 90 degrees = −1
- 90 degrees = 0
- 60 degrees = 1
- 45 degrees = 2
- 30 degrees = 3
- 0 degrees = 4

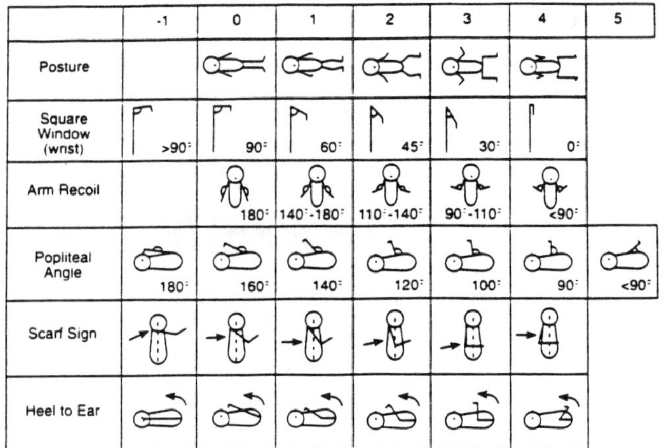

FIGURE II.1. Neuromuscular maturity. (Modified from Ballard JL, Khoury JC, Wedig K, et al. New Ballard score, expanded to include extremely premature infants. *J Pediatr* 1991; 119:417–423; and Dubowitz LM, Dubowitz V, Goldberg C. Clinical assessment of gestational age in the newborn infant. *J Pediatr* 1970; 77:1–10, with permission.)

Arm Recoil

With the infant supine, fully flex the forearm for 5 seconds and then fully extend it by pulling the hands and release. Score the reaction as follows:

- Remains extended 180 degrees or random movements = 0
- Minimal flexion, 140 to 180 degrees = 1
- Small amount of flexion, 110 to 140 degrees = 2
- Moderate flexion, 90 to 100 degrees = 3
- Brisk return to full flexion, less than 90 degrees = 4

Popliteal Angle

With the infant supine and the pelvis flat on the examining surface, the leg is flexed on the thigh and the thigh fully flexed with one hand. With the other hand, the leg is then extended and the angle is scored according to the following:

- 180 degrees = −1
- 160 degrees = 0

- 140 degrees = 1
- 120 degrees = 2
- 100 degrees = 3
- 90 degrees = 4
- Less than 90 degrees = 5

Scarf Sign

With the infant supine, take the infant's hand and draw it across the neck and as far across the opposite shoulder as possible. Assistance to the elbow is permissible by lifting it across the body. Score according to the location of the elbow as follows:

- Elbow reaches or nears the level of opposite shoulder = –1
- Elbow crosses the opposite anterior axillary line = 0
- Elbow reaches the opposite anterior axillary line = 1
- Elbow is at midline = 2
- Elbow does not reach midline = 3
- Elbow does not cross the proximate axillary line = 4

Heel to Ear

With the infant supine, hold the infant's foot with one hand and move it as near to the head as possible without forcing it. Keep the pelvis flat on the examining surface. Score as shown in the Fig. II.1.

Physical Maturity

See Table II.1 for information for scoring physical maturity.

Maturity Rating

Add up the individual Neuromuscular and Physical Maturity scores for the 12 categories and then obtain the estimated gestational age from Tables II.1 and II.2.

CLASSIFICATION OF NEWBORNS BASED ON MATURITY AND INTRAUTERINE GROWTH

See Fig. II.2 for classification.

TABLE II.1 Physical Maturity

Sign	−1	0	1	2	3	4	5
Skin	Sticky, friable, transparent	Gelatinous red, translucent	Smooth pink, visible veins	Superficial peeling and/or rash, few veins	Cracking, pale areas, rare veins	Parchment, deep cracking, no vessels	Leathery, cracked, wrinkled
Lanugo	None	Sparse	Abundant	Thinning	Bald areas	Mostly bald	—
Plantar creases	Heel to toe, 40–50 mm = −1; <40 mm = −2	Heel to toe >50 mm, no creases	Faint red marks	Anterior transverse crease only	Creases over anterior two-thirds	Creases over entire sole	—
Breast	Imperceptible	Barely perceptible	Flat areola, no bud	Stippled areola, 1–2 mm bud	Raised areola, 3–4 mm bud	Full areola, 5–10 mm bud	—

Eye and ear	Lids fused, loosely = –1; tightly = –2	Lids open, pinna flat, stays folded	Slightly curved pinna, soft with slow recoil	Well-curved pinna, soft but ready recoil	Formed and firm, with instant recoil	Thick cartilage, ear stiff	—
Genitals, male	Scrotum flat, smooth	Scrotum empty, faint rugae	Testes in upper canal, rare rugae	Testes descending, few rugae	Testes down, good rugae	Testes pendulous, deep rugae	—
Genitals, female	Clitoris prominent, labia flat	Prominent clitoris, small labia minora	Prominent clitoris, enlarging minora	Majora and minora equally prominent	Majora large, minora small	Majora cover clitoris and minora	—

Modified from Ballard JL, Khoury JC, Wedig K, et al. New Ballard score, expanded to include extremely premature infants. *J Pediatr* 1991; 119:417–423; and Dubowitz LM, Dubowitz V, Goldberg C. Clinical assessment of gestational age in the newborn infant. *J Pediatr* 1970; 77:1–10, with permission.

TABLE II.2 Maturity Rating

Total Score	Gestational Age (wk)
–10	20
–5	22
0	24
5	26
10	28
15	30
20	32
25	34
30	36
35	38
40	40
45	42
50	44

Modified from Ballard JL, Khoury JC, Wedig K, et al. New Ballard score, expanded to include extremely premature infants. *J Pediatr* 1991; 119:417–423; and Dubowitz LM, Dubowitz V, Goldberg C. Clinical assessment of gestational age in the newborn infant. *J Pediatr* 1970; 77:1–10, with permission.

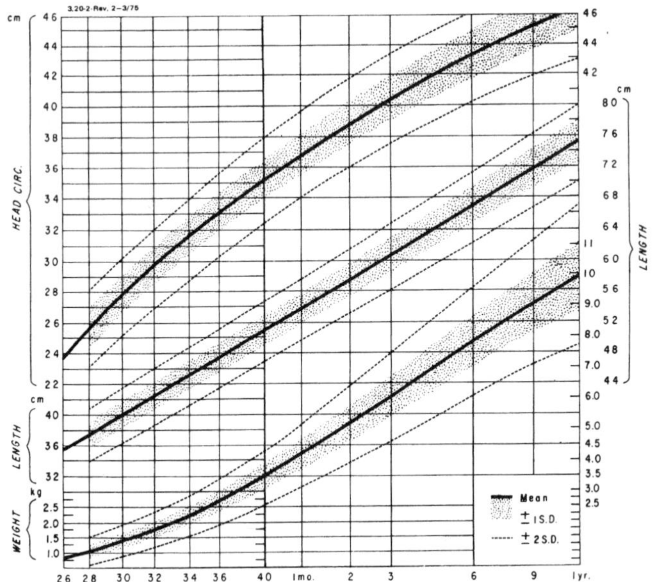

FIGURE II.2. A fetal-infant growth graph for infants varying in gestational ages. (From Dr. S. G. Babson, Department of Pediatrics, University of Oregon School of Medicine, Portland, Oregon, with permission.)

Suggested Reading

Ballard JL, Khoury JC, Wedig K, et al. New Ballard score, expanded to include extremely premature infants. *J Pediatr* 1991;119:417–423.

Ballard JL, Novak KK, Driver M. A simplified score for assessment of fetal maturation of newly born infants. *J Pediatr* 1979;95:769–774.

Dubowitz LM, Dubowitz V, Goldberg C. Clinical assessment of gestational age in the newborn infant. *J Pediatr* 1970;77:1–10.

Klaus MH, Fanaroff AA, eds. *Care of the high-risk neonate,* 3rd ed. Philadelphia: WB Saunders, 1986: 80–83.

Appendix III

Head Circumference for Age Percentiles

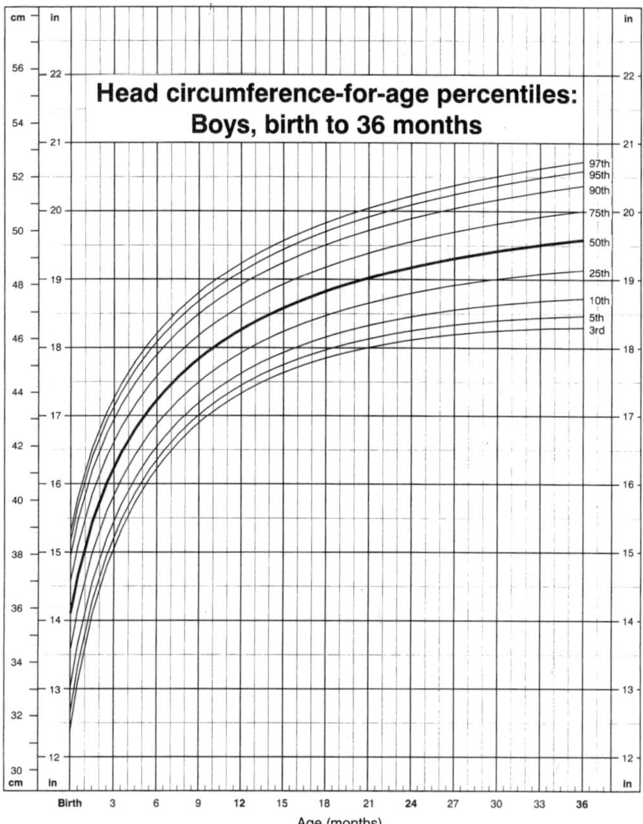

FIGURE III.1. Head circumference for age percentiles. (From the National Center for Health Statistics in collaboration with the National Center for Chronic Disease Prevention and Health Promotion (2000). Centers for Disease Control and Prevention website. Available at: *http://www.cdc.gov/growthcharts/.* Accessed December 10, 2002, with permission.)

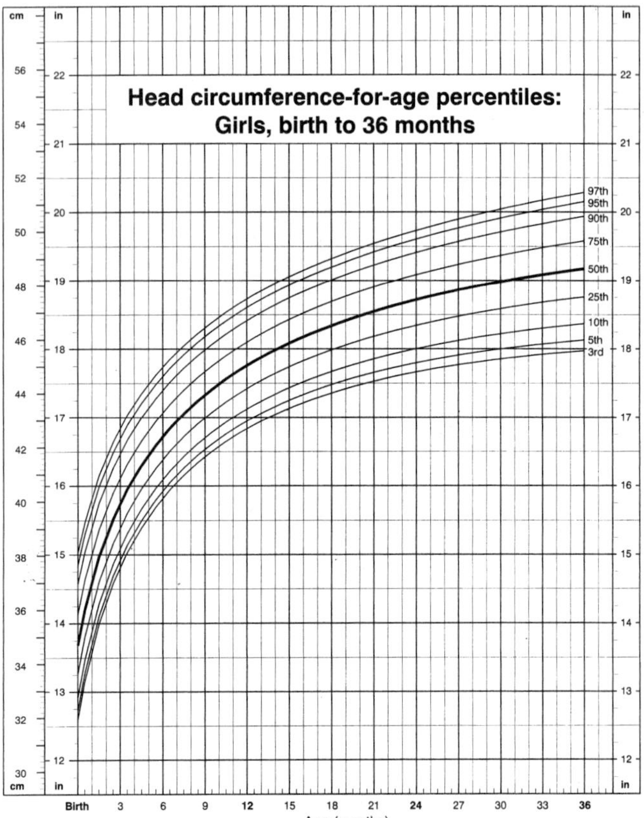

FIGURE III.2. Head circumference for age percentiles. (From the National Center for Health Statistics in collaboration with the National Center for Chronic Disease Prevention and Health Promotion (2000). Centers for Disease Control and Prevention website. Available at: *http://www.cdc.gov/growthcharts/.* Accessed December 10, 2002, with permission.)

Appendix IV

Age of Copying Figures

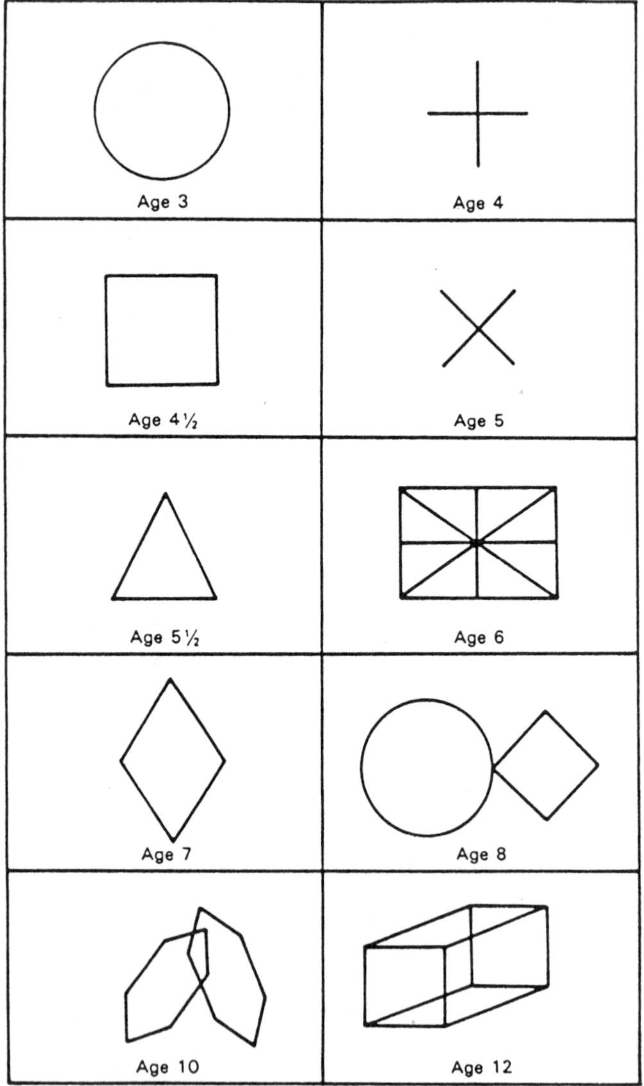

FIGURE IV.1. Approximate age at which a child can copy figures.

Appendix V

Apgar Score

TABLE V.1 Apgar Score

Signs	0	1	2
Heart rate	Absent	Below 100	Over 100
Respiratory effect	Absent	Slow, irregular	Good, crying
Muscle tone	Limp	Some flexion of extremities	Active motion
Response to catheter in nostril (tested after oropharynx is clear)	No response	Grimace	Cough or sneeze
Color	Blue, pale	Body pink, extremities blue	Complete pink

Sixty seconds after the complete birth of the infant (disregard the cord and placenta) the five objective signs above are evaluated, and each is given a score of 0, 1, or 2. A total score of 10 indicates an infant in the best possible condition.

From Apgar V. Proposal for new method of evaluation of newborn infant. *Anesthesia and Analgesia.* 1953;32:260–267, with permission.

Appendix VI

Glasgow Coma Scale

TABLE VI.1 Glasgow Coma Scale

Category	Score
Eyes open	
Never	1
To pain	2
To verbal stimuli	3
Spontaneously	4
Best verbal response	
None	1
Incomprehensible	2
Inappropriate words	3
Disoriented, conversing	4
Oriented, conversing	5
Best motor response	
None	1
Extension	2
Flexion abnormal	3
Flexion withdrawal	4
Localizing pain	5
Obeys commands	6
Total	15

From Teasdale G, Jennet B. Assessment of coma and impaired consciousness: a practical scale. *Lancet* 1974;2:81–84, with permission.

Appendix VII

Management of Concussion

TABLE VII.1 Grades of Concussion

Grade 1	Grade 2	Grade 3
1. Transient confusion (inattention, inability to maintain a coherent stream of thought and to carry out goal-directed movements) 2. No loss of consciousness 3. Concussion symptoms or mental status abnormalities on examination resolve in less than 15 min	1. Transient confusion 2. No loss of consciousness 3. Concussion symptoms or mental status abnormalities (including amnesia) on examination last **more than 15 min**	1. Any loss of consciousness: a. Brief (sec) b. Prolonged (min)

From Quality Standards Subcommittee of the American Academy of Neurology. The management of concussion in sports [practice parameter]. *Neurology* 1997;48:581–585, with permission.

TABLE VII.2 Management Recommendations

Grade 1	Grade 2	Grade 3
1. Remove from contest. 2. Examine immediately and at 5-min intervals for the development of mental status abnormalities or postconcussive symptoms at rest with exertion. 3. May return to contest if mental status abnormalities or postconcussive symptoms clear within 15 min.	1. Remove from contest and disallow return that day. 2. Examine on-site frequently for signs of evolving intracranial pathology. 3. A trained person should reexamine the athlete the following day. 4. A physician should perform a neurologic examination to clear the athlete for return to play after one full asymptomatic week at rest and with exertion.	1. Transport the athlete from the field to the nearest emergency department by ambulance if still unconscious or if worrisome signs are detected (with cervical spine immobilization, if indicated). 2. A thorough neurologic evaluation should be performed emergently, including appropriate neuroimaging procedures when indicated. 3. Hospital admission is indicated if signs of pathology are detected or if the mental status of the athlete remains abnormal.

From Quality Standards Subcommittee of the American Academy of Neurology. The management of concussion in sports [practice parameter]. *Neurology* 1997;48:581–585, with permission.

TABLE VII.3 When to Return to Play After Concussion

Grade of Concussion	Return to Play Only After Being Asymptomatic With Normal Neurologic Assessment at Rest and With Exercise
Grade 1 concussion	15 min or less
Multiple grade 1 concussions	1 wk
Grade 2 concussion	1 wk
Multiple grade 2 concussions	2 wk
Grade 3—brief loss of consciousness (sec)	1 wk
Grade 3—prolonged loss of consciousness (min)	2 wk
Multiple grade 3 concussions	1 month or longer, based on decision of evaluating physician

From Quality Standards Subcommittee of the American Academy of Neurology. The management of concussion in sports [practice parameter]. *Neurology* 1997;48:581–585, with permission.

TABLE VII.4 Features of Concussion Frequently Observed

1. Vacant stare (befuddled facial expression)
2. Delayed verbal and motor responses (slow to answer questions or follow instructions)
3. Confusion and inability to focus attention (easily distracted and unable to follow through with normal activities)
4. Disorientation (walking in the wrong direction; unaware of time, date, and place)
5. Slurred or incoherent speech (making disjointed or incomprehensible statements)
6. Gross observable incoordination (stumbling, inability to walk tandem or in a straight line)
7. Emotions out of proportion to circumstances (distraught, crying for no apparent reason)
8. Memory deficits (exhibited by the athlete repeatedly asking the same question that has already been answered or inability to memorize or recall three of three words or three of three objects in 5 min)
9. Any period of loss of consciousness (paralytic coma, unresponsiveness to arousal)

From Quality Standards Subcommittee of the American Academy of Neurology. The management of concussion in sports [practice parameter]. *Neurology* 1997;48:581–585, with permission.

TABLE VII.5 Sideline Evaluation

Mental status testing

Orientation:	Time, place, person, and situation (circumstances of injury)
Concentration:	Digits backward (i.e., 3–1–7, 4–6–8–2, 5–3–0–7–4) Months of the year in reverse order
Memory:	Names of teams in prior contest Recall of three words and three objects at 0 and 5 min Recent newsworthy events Details of the contest (e.g., plays, moves, strategies)

Exertional Provocative Tests	Neurologic Tests
40-yard sprint	Strength
5 push-ups	Coordination and agility
5 sit-ups	Sensation
5 knee-bends	

From Quality Standards Subcommittee of the American Academy of Neurology. The management of concussion in sports [practice parameter]. *Neurology* 1997;48:581–585, with permission.

Appendix VIII

Commonly Used Drugs in Neurology

Generic Name	*Dose*
Anticonvulsants	
Carbamazepine	10–40 mg/kg/d
Clonazepam	0.1–0.2 mg/kg/d
Diazepam	0.3–0.5 mg/kg/dose (intravenous [i.v.])
Ethosuximide	10–40 mg/kg/d
Felbamate	15–45 mg/kg/d
Fosphenytoin	10–20 mg/kg of phenytoin equivalents
Gabapentin*	15–40 mg/kg/d
Lamotrigine	1–5 mg/kg/d with valproate (maintenance)
	5–15 mg/kg/day without valproate, up to 400 mg/kg/d (maintenance)
Levetiracetam*	20–40 mg/kg (maintenance)
Lorazepam	0.05–0.1 mg/kg/d; 1–4 mg i.v.
Mysoline	10–40 mg/kg/d
Oxcarbazepine	8–10 mg/kg/d, maximum 1,200–1,800 mg/kg/day; 20–50 mg/kg/d (maintenance)
Phenobarbitol	3–7 mg/kg/d up to 30 kg, then 60 mg twice daily (b.i.d.)
Phenytoin	5–10 mg/kg/d, maximum of 300 mg/kg/day
Tiagabine*	4–32 mg/d

*Not approved for children. Please refer to Table 17.2 for United States Food and Drug Administration (FDA)-approved indications for newer antiepileptic drugs.

Topiramate	5–9 mg/kg/d (maintenance)
Valproic acid	10–60 mg/kg/d
Zonisamide*	4–8 mg/kg (maintenance)

Condition	*Drug category*	*Drug*	*Pediatric Dose*
Headache			
		Acetaminophen	10–15 mg/kg every 6–8 h
		Amitriptyline	1–3 mg/kg/d
		Carbamazepine	10–40 mg/kg/d
		Cyproheptadine	0.25 mg/kg b.i.d., maximum of 12 mg
		Fiorinal	Compound drug; dose not established for children
		Gabapentin	15–40 mg/kg/d
		Ibuprofen	4–10 mg/kg every 6–8 h
		Propanolol	0.6–1.5 mg/kg/d, maximum 4 mg/kg/d
		Rizatriptan	Not established for children under 12 years of age
		Sumatriptan	Not established for children under

*Not approved for children. Please refer to Table 17.2 for United States Food and Drug Administration (FDA)-approved indications for newer antiepileptic drugs.

		12 years of age
	Valproic acid	10–60 mg/kg/d
	Verapamil	Not established for children under 12 years of age
	Zolmitriptan	Not established for children under 12 years of age
Stimulants		
	Adderall	2.5–40 mg/d for children over 6 yr of age; for those 3 to 5 yr of age, 2.5 mg/d
	Concerta	18–54 mg/d for children over 6 yr of age
	Dexedrine	5–40 mg/d for children over 6 yr of age; for those 3 to 6 yr of age, 2.5–40 mg/d
	Methylphenidate	0.3 to 2 mg/kg/d b.i.d. for those over 6 yr of age; maximum 60 mg

			Usual dose 5–15 mg b.i.d.
	Selected psychiatric drugs		
		Selective serotonin reuptake inhibitors	
		Citalopram	Not established for children under 12 years of age
		Fluoxetine	5–20 mg/d for children over 5 yr of age
		Paroxetine	10–30 mg/d for children over 8 yr of age
		Sertraline	25–200 mg/d for those 6 to 12 yr of age
		Tricyclics	
		Amitriptyline	1–3 mg/kg/d
		Clomipramine	Not established for children under 12 years of age
		Imipramine	1.5–5 mg/kg/d
Myasthenia gravis			
		Neostigmine	2 mg/kg/d orally (p.o.) 0.01–0.04 mg/kg, intra-

		muscular (i.m.), i.v., subcutaneously (s.c.)
	Pyridostigmine	Titer dose for effect, 7 mg/kg/d in 5–6 divided doses
		2 mg i.m. or i.v. every 2–3 h
	Tensilon	0.1 mg/kg i.v., up to 10 mg; have atropine available
Sedatives		
	Chloral hydrate	25 mg/kg/dose, sedative
		50 mg/kg/dose, soporific
		75 mg/kg/dose, anesthetic
	Diphenhydramine	5 mg/kg/dose
Impulse control disorders		
	Haloperidol	0.01–0.03 mg/kg/d for those 3 to 12 yr of age (titer for effect)
	Thioridazine	10–100 mg/d for those over 2 yr of age (titer for effect)

Steroids		
	Cortisone	25–30 mg/m², physiologic 75–100 mg/m², stress dose more than 100 mg/m², pharmacologic
	Dexamethasone	12 mg/m²
	Prednisone	0.5–2 mg/kg/d
Muscle relaxants		
	Baclofen	5–20 mg three times a day (t.i.d.)
	Dantrolene	6 mg/kg/d
	Methocarbamol	Not established for children under 12 years of age
Intravenous immunoglobulin		0.4 mg/kg/d for 5 days i.v. **OR** 1 g/kg/d for 2 days i.v.

Appendix IX

Differential Diagnoses

Long lists of differential diagnoses are generally unhelpful. This handbook is meant to be comprehensive and nonencyclopedic. What follows are selected topics that may provide the reader with a starting point for evaluating disease processes. Not all processes mentioned in these lists can be found in the handbook. Rather, they are provided to initiate a more thorough search for the underlying treatment and cause of a presenting complaint.

ATAXIA

- Developmental
- Drug intoxication
- Metabolic abnormalities
- Brain tumors
- Infection
- Hereditary
- Paraneoplastic

BACK PAIN

- Trauma
- Developmental
- Root pain
- Inflammatory
- Discogenic

BEHAVIOR DISTURBANCE

- Pervasive developmental disorders
- Autism
- Asperger syndrome
- Attention deficit hyperactivity disorder
- Conduct disorder
- Obsessive-compulsive disorder
- Oppositional defiant syndromes

COMA

- Drugs
- Increased intracranial pressure
- Metabolic (e.g., diabetes, renal or liver disease)
- Infection
- Seizure
- Hypoxic-ischemic events
- Trauma

CRANIAL NEUROPATHIES

- Optic nerve
  - Demyelinating
  - Devic disease
  - Tumor
  - Hereditary
- Cavernous sinus infection or thrombosis (cranial nerves III, IV, and VI and V-1, V-2)
- Infantile botulism (III)
- Myasthenia (III, IV, VI)
- Diabetes (III)
- Brainstem tumor (III, VI, VII, bulbar nerves)
- Duane syndrome (VI)
- Möbius syndrome (VI, VII)
- Petrous apicitis (VI, VII)
- Nonspecific sign of increased intracranial pressure (VI)
- Myopathy (oculopharyngeal)
- Kearns-Sayres (external ophthalmoplegia)
- Cerebellar pontine angle (V, VII, VIII)

HEMIPARESIS

- Stroke
- Seizures
- Trauma
- Vasculitis
- Encephalitis
- Migraine
- Vascular malformations
- Tumor
- Dissection

INCREASED INTRACRANIAL PRESSURE

- Meningitis
- Tumor
- Encephalitis
- Hemorrhage
- Abscess
- Pseudotumor cerebri

INFECTIOUS DISEASE

- Bacterial
- Viral
- Fungal
- Parainfectious
- Human immunodeficiency virus
- Intrauterine infection other than TORCH
- Toxoplasmosis, rubella, cytomegalovirus, and herpes simplex ("TORCH" infections)

INTRACRANIAL MASS

- Subdural hematoma
- Brain abscess
- Brain tumors
- Cortical dysplasia
- Mitochondrial encephalomyopathy, lactic acidemia, and stroke-like episodes (MELAS)
- Coagulopathies (proteins C and S, antithrombin III, Leiden factor, and phospholipid antibodies)

LEUKEMIA: NEUROLOGIC COMPLICATIONS

- Leptomeningeal metastases
- Hydrocephalus
- Cranial neuropathies
- Cerebrovascular accident(CVA)
- Hypothalamic syndrome
- Infection
- Spinal cord compression
- Neuropathy

MACROCEPHALY

- Familial
- Storage disease
- Hydrocephalus
- Brain tumor
- Genetic
  - Neurofibromatosis
  - Achondroplasia
  - Hurler syndrome

MENTAL RETARDATION

Static

- Hypoxic-ischemic injury
- Intraventricular hemorrhage
- Intrauterine infection (TORCH infections)
- Intrauterine toxins (alcohol, smoking, drugs)
- Developmental disorders: disorders of induction, migration, proliferation, and organization
- Trauma
- Genetic
- Idiopathic

Progressive (Dementia)

- Inborn errors of metabolism
  - Aminoacidopathies
  - Organicacidemia
- Lysosomal disorders
- Peroxisomal disorders

- Mucopolysaccharidosis
- Ceroid lipofuscinosis
- Brain tumors
- Hallervorden-Spatz disease
- Wilson disease
- Menkes disease
- Mitochondrial disorders
- Toxins (radiation, chemotherapy)

MICROCEPHALY

- Intrauterine infection
- Genetic
- Intrauterine exposure to drugs
- Developmental disorder
- Degenerative disease (e.g., Rett syndrome)
- Craniosynostosis

MOVEMENT DISORDERS

- Myoclonus
  - Anoxia
  - Seizures
  - Degenerative disease
  - Metabolic
- Tics and tremors
  - Infection
  - Hereditary
  - Tourette syndrome
- Choreoathetosis
  - Sydenham chorea
  - Huntington chorea
  - Carbon monoxide exposure
  - Lupus
  - Pregnancy
- Paroxysmal choreoathetosis
- Paroxysmal ataxia

MUSCLE DISEASE

- Congenital myopathies
- Muscular dystrophies

- Myotonic dystrophies
- Metabolic: acid maltase deficiency
- Inflammatory
- Neuromuscular junction disorders
  - Myasthenia
  - Botulism
- Periodic paralysis

NEOPLASIA: NEUROLOGIC COMPLICATIONS OF TREATMENT

- Endocrinopathies
- Dementia
- Leukoencephalopathy
- Seizures
- Secondary oncogenesis

NEUROCUTANEOUS SYNDROMES (MOST COMMON)

- Neurofibromatosis
- von Hippel-Lindau syndrome
- Tuberous sclerosis
- Sturge-Weber (trigeminal encephaloangiomatosis)
- Ataxia telangiectasis
- Incontinentia pigmenti
- Linea nevus syndromes

NEUROPATHIES

Acute

- Trauma
- Inflammatory: appears after infections
  - Guillain-Barré syndrome
  - Chronic inflammatory demyelinating polyradiculoneuropathy (CIDP)
- Infectious
  - Cranial nerve VI
  - Cranial nerve VII (Bell palsy)
- Brachial plexitis
  - Brachial plexus injury in newborn
  - Idiopathic
  - Hereditary

Chronic

- Hereditary
  - Sensory-motor neuropathies
  - Refsum disease
- Degenerative
- Metabolic
  - Diabetic
  - Sarcoid
  - Autoimmune

PTOSIS

- Congenital
- Oculomotor paresis
- Ophthalmoplegic migraine
- Myasthenia gravis
- Carotid artery dissection

SEIZURES

- Generalized
- Simple partial
- Complete partial
- Neonatal seizures
- Infantile spasms

SPINAL CORD DISEASE

- Trauma: spinal cord injury without radiographic abnormality (SCIWORA)
- Compressive disease
  - Blood
  - Pus
  - Tumor
- Developmental
  - Tethered cord
  - Diplomyelia
  - Diastematomyelia
  - Syringomyelia
  - Lipoma

- Infectious
  - Demyelinating
  - Transverse myelitis
  - Discitis
- Arteriovenous malformation (AVM)

SYNCOPE

- Vasovagal
- Cardiac
- Metabolic (e.g., diabetes)
- Cerebrovascular
- Seizure
- Anxiety

Subject Index

Note: Page numbers followed by *f* indicate figures; those followed by *t* indicate tables.

M